This notebook belongs to:

_____

Published by: Character Designs

30 DAY
WATER
challenge

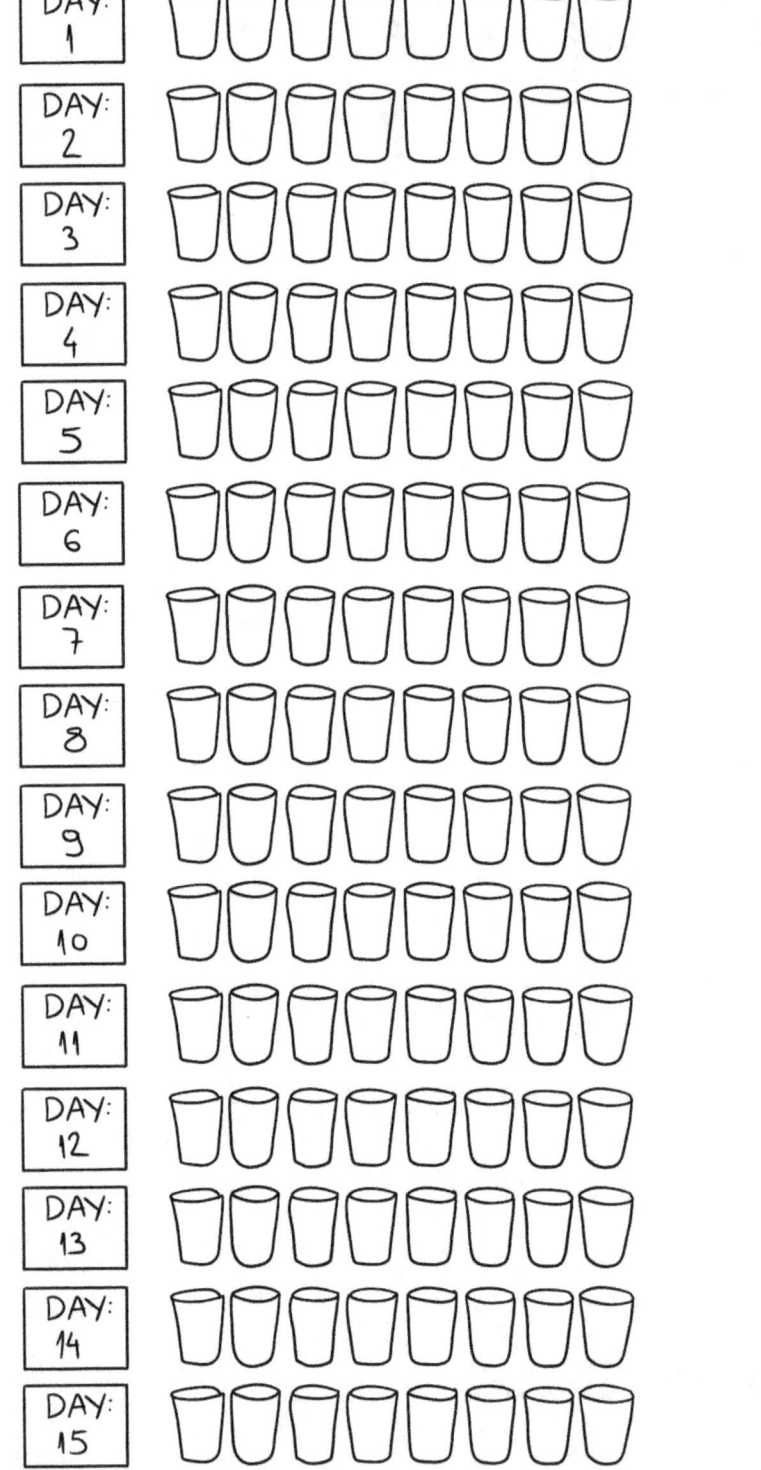

DAY: 1								
DAY: 2								
DAY: 3								
DAY: 4								
DAY: 5								
DAY: 6								
DAY: 7								
DAY: 8								
DAY: 9								
DAY: 10								
DAY: 11								
DAY: 12								
DAY: 13								
DAY: 14								
DAY: 15								
DAY: 16								
DAY: 17								
DAY: 18								
DAY: 19								
DAY: 20								
DAY: 21								
DAY: 22								
DAY: 23								
DAY: 24								
DAY: 25								
DAY: 26								
DAY: 27								
DAY: 28								
DAY: 29								
DAY: 30								

30 DAY
WATER
challenge

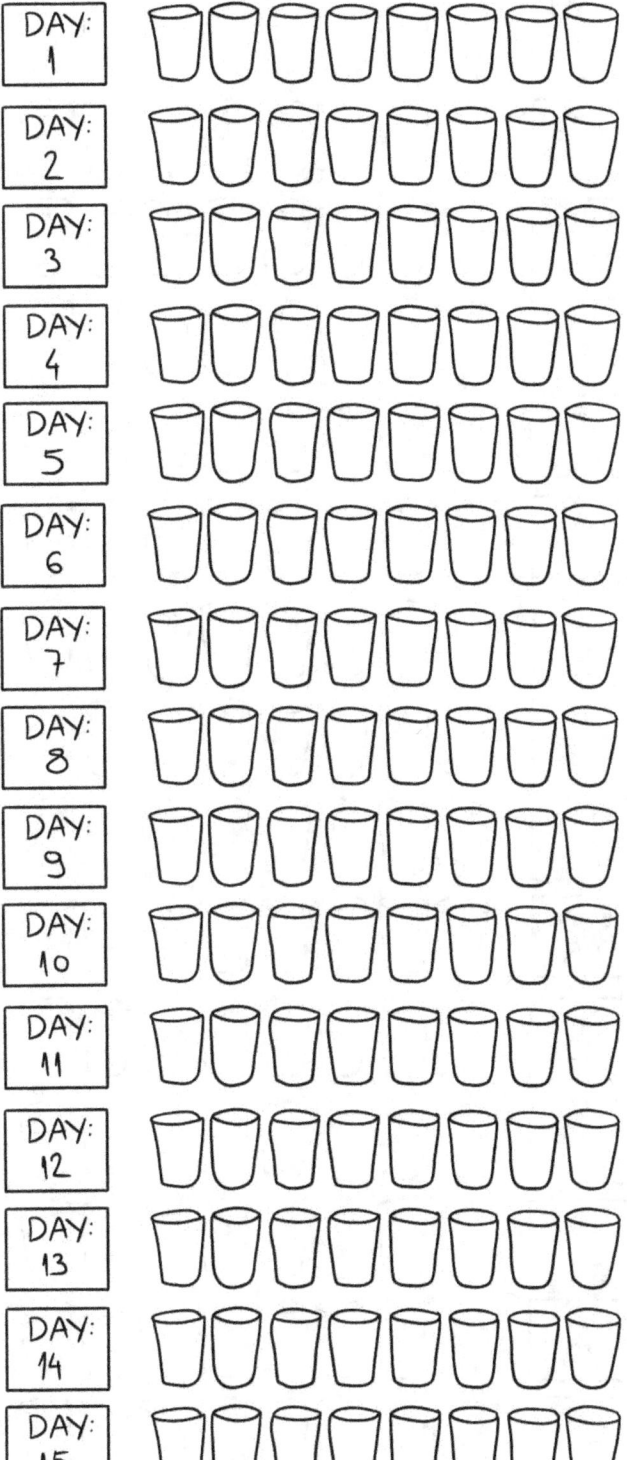

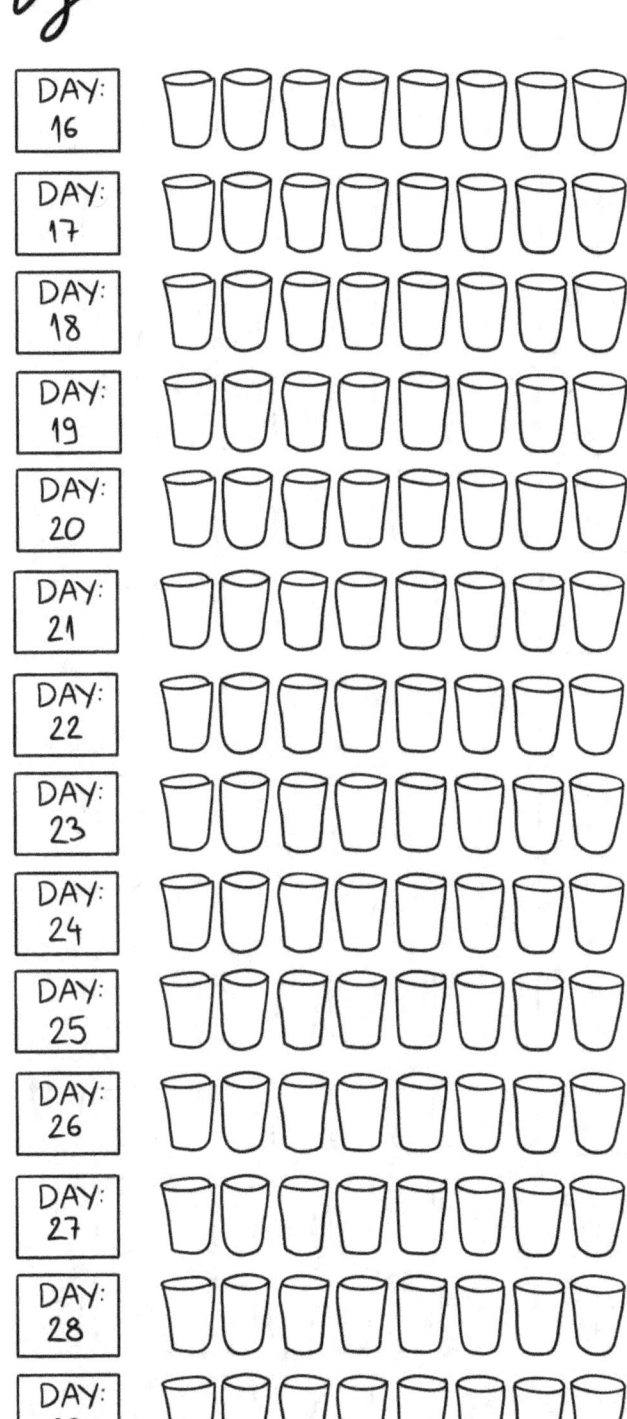

30 DAY
WATER
challenge

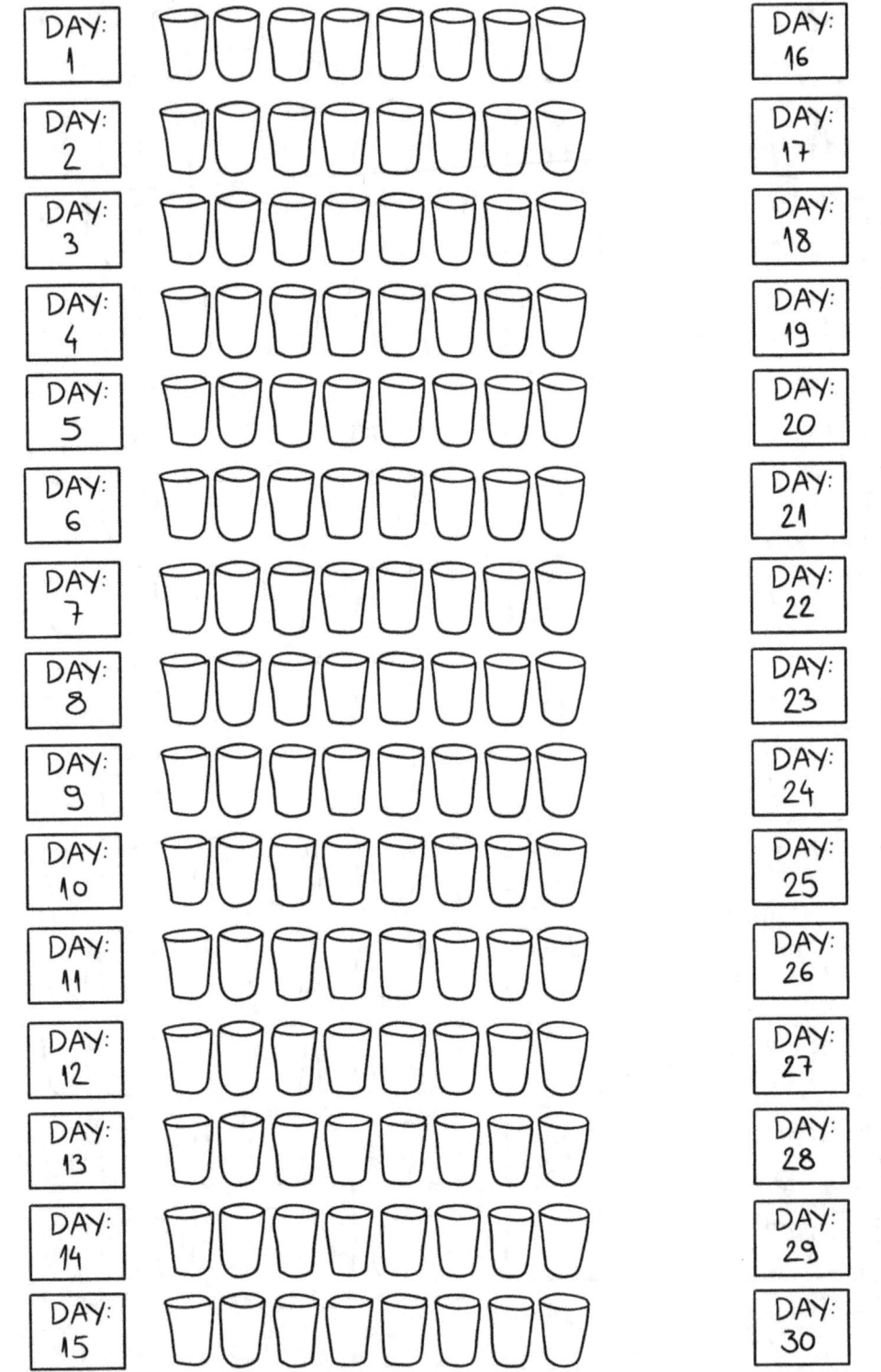

DAY: 1							
DAY: 2							
DAY: 3							
DAY: 4							
DAY: 5							
DAY: 6							
DAY: 7							
DAY: 8							
DAY: 9							
DAY: 10							
DAY: 11							
DAY: 12							
DAY: 13							
DAY: 14							
DAY: 15							

DAY: 16							
DAY: 17							
DAY: 18							
DAY: 19							
DAY: 20							
DAY: 21							
DAY: 22							
DAY: 23							
DAY: 24							
DAY: 25							
DAY: 26							
DAY: 27							
DAY: 28							
DAY: 29							
DAY: 30							

30 DAY
WATER
challenge

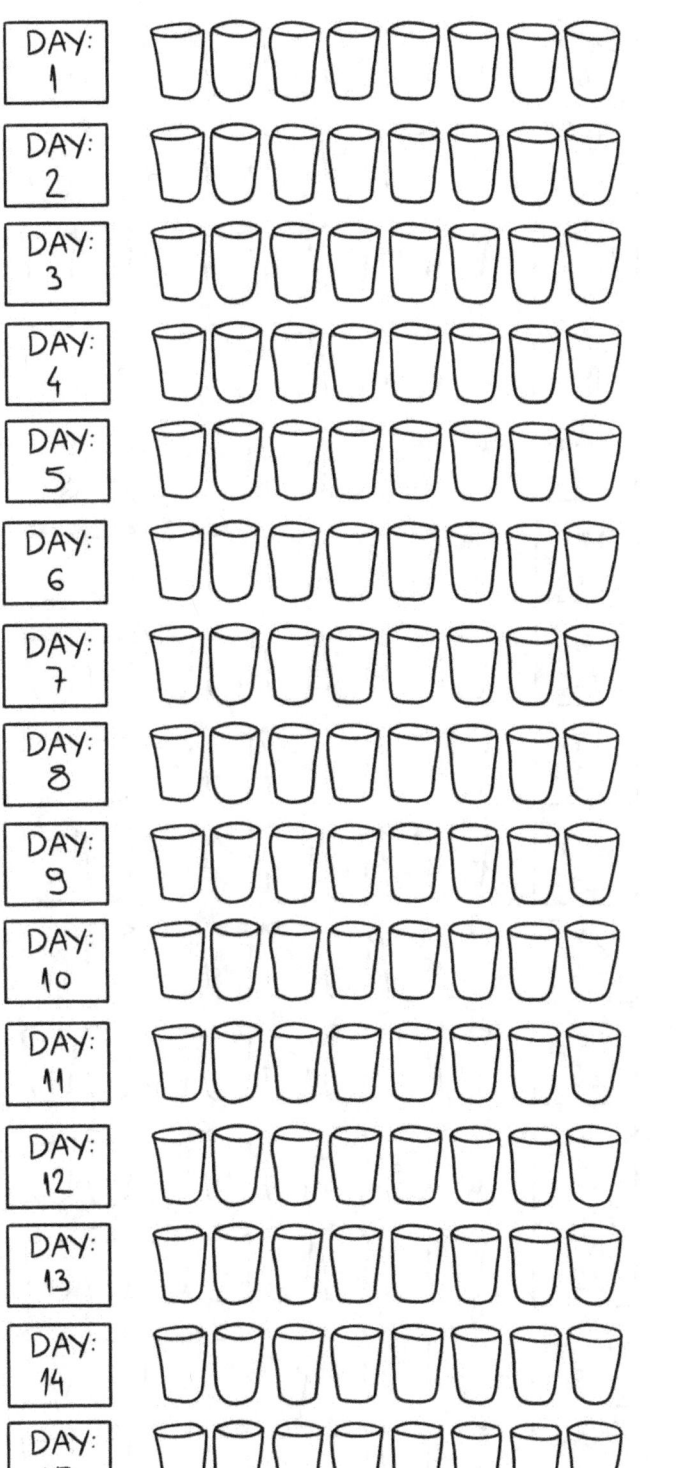

DAY: 1		DAY: 16
DAY: 2		DAY: 17
DAY: 3		DAY: 18
DAY: 4		DAY: 19
DAY: 5		DAY: 20
DAY: 6		DAY: 21
DAY: 7		DAY: 22
DAY: 8		DAY: 23
DAY: 9		DAY: 24
DAY: 10		DAY: 25
DAY: 11		DAY: 26
DAY: 12		DAY: 27
DAY: 13		DAY: 28
DAY: 14		DAY: 29
DAY: 15		DAY: 30

30 DAY
WATER
challenge

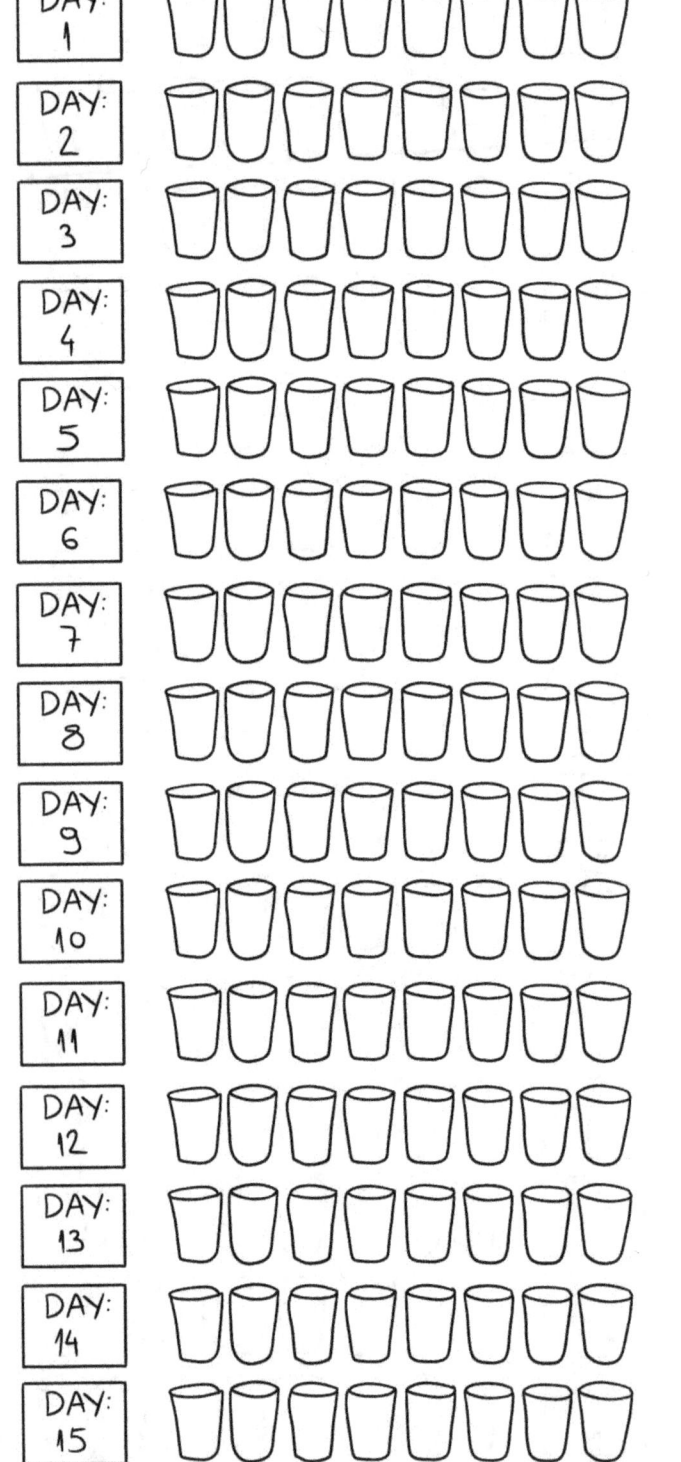

DAY: 1	DAY: 16
DAY: 2	DAY: 17
DAY: 3	DAY: 18
DAY: 4	DAY: 19
DAY: 5	DAY: 20
DAY: 6	DAY: 21
DAY: 7	DAY: 22
DAY: 8	DAY: 23
DAY: 9	DAY: 24
DAY: 10	DAY: 25
DAY: 11	DAY: 26
DAY: 12	DAY: 27
DAY: 13	DAY: 28
DAY: 14	DAY: 29
DAY: 15	DAY: 30

30 DAY
WATER
challenge

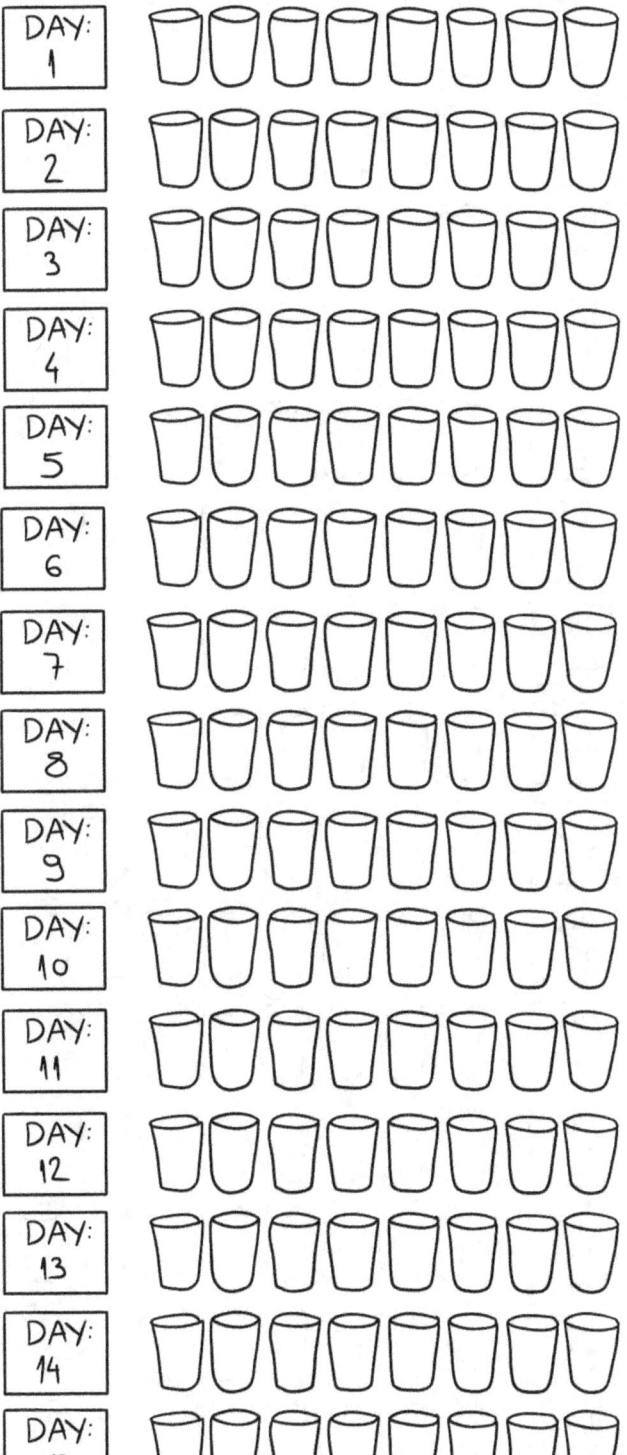

DAY: 1	⌒⌒⌒⌒⌒⌒⌒⌒
DAY: 2	⌒⌒⌒⌒⌒⌒⌒⌒
DAY: 3	⌒⌒⌒⌒⌒⌒⌒⌒
DAY: 4	⌒⌒⌒⌒⌒⌒⌒⌒
DAY: 5	⌒⌒⌒⌒⌒⌒⌒⌒
DAY: 6	⌒⌒⌒⌒⌒⌒⌒⌒
DAY: 7	⌒⌒⌒⌒⌒⌒⌒⌒
DAY: 8	⌒⌒⌒⌒⌒⌒⌒⌒
DAY: 9	⌒⌒⌒⌒⌒⌒⌒⌒
DAY: 10	⌒⌒⌒⌒⌒⌒⌒⌒
DAY: 11	⌒⌒⌒⌒⌒⌒⌒⌒
DAY: 12	⌒⌒⌒⌒⌒⌒⌒⌒
DAY: 13	⌒⌒⌒⌒⌒⌒⌒⌒
DAY: 14	⌒⌒⌒⌒⌒⌒⌒⌒
DAY: 15	⌒⌒⌒⌒⌒⌒⌒⌒

DAY: 16	⌒⌒⌒⌒⌒⌒⌒⌒
DAY: 17	⌒⌒⌒⌒⌒⌒⌒⌒
DAY: 18	⌒⌒⌒⌒⌒⌒⌒⌒
DAY: 19	⌒⌒⌒⌒⌒⌒⌒⌒
DAY: 20	⌒⌒⌒⌒⌒⌒⌒⌒
DAY: 21	⌒⌒⌒⌒⌒⌒⌒⌒
DAY: 22	⌒⌒⌒⌒⌒⌒⌒⌒
DAY: 23	⌒⌒⌒⌒⌒⌒⌒⌒
DAY: 24	⌒⌒⌒⌒⌒⌒⌒⌒
DAY: 25	⌒⌒⌒⌒⌒⌒⌒⌒
DAY: 26	⌒⌒⌒⌒⌒⌒⌒⌒
DAY: 27	⌒⌒⌒⌒⌒⌒⌒⌒
DAY: 28	⌒⌒⌒⌒⌒⌒⌒⌒
DAY: 29	⌒⌒⌒⌒⌒⌒⌒⌒
DAY: 30	⌒⌒⌒⌒⌒⌒⌒⌒

30 DAY
WATER
challenge

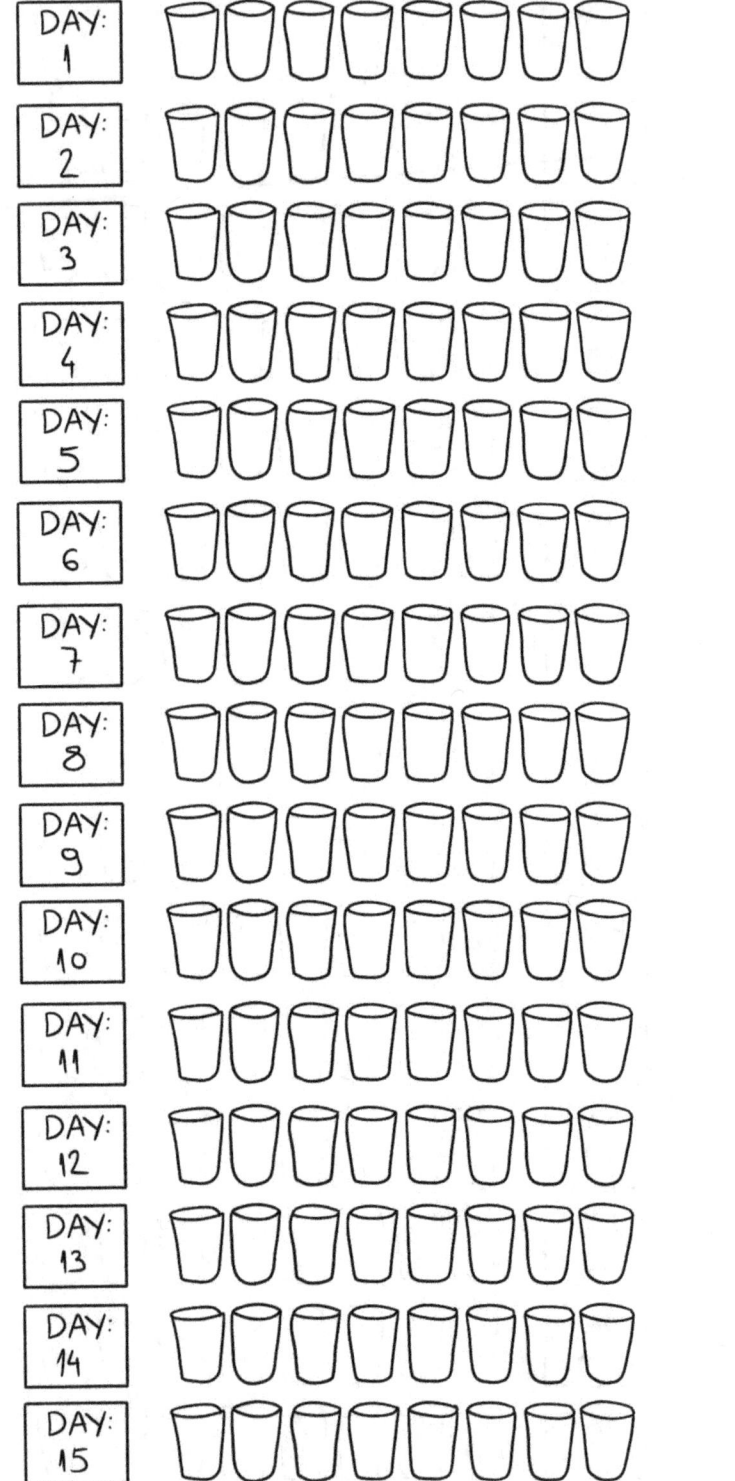

30 DAY
WATER
challenge

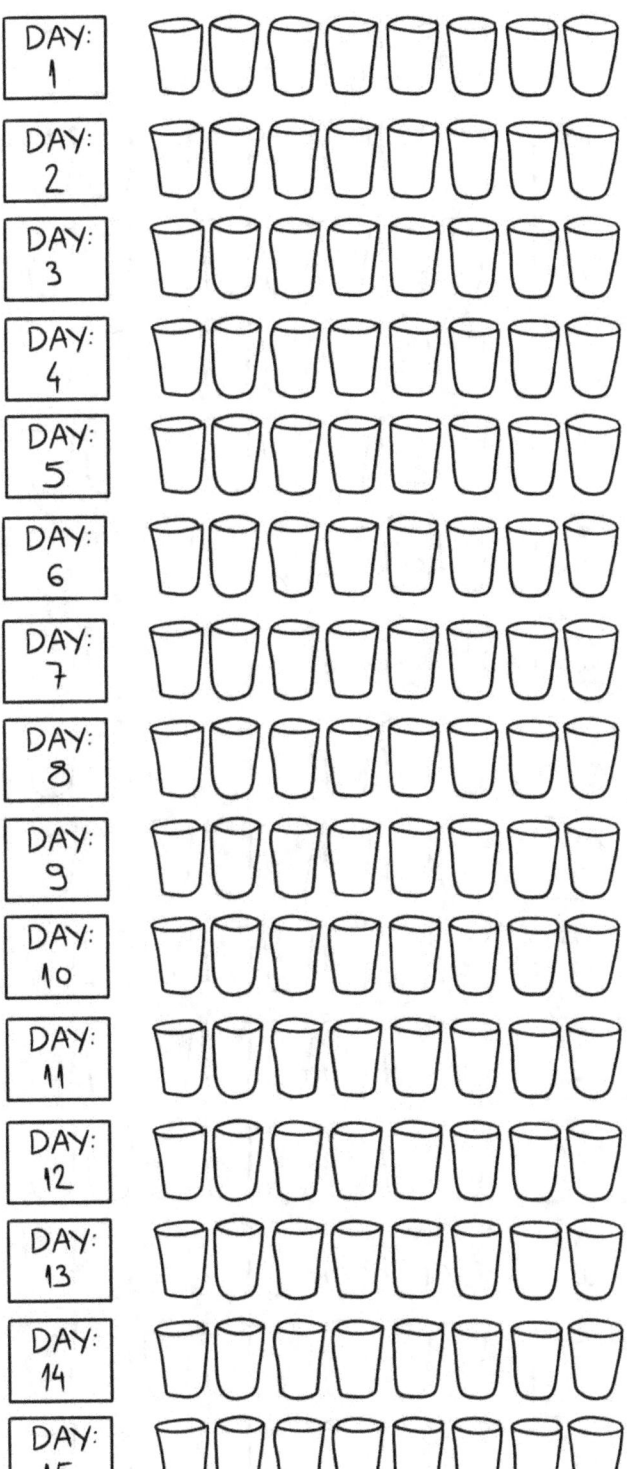

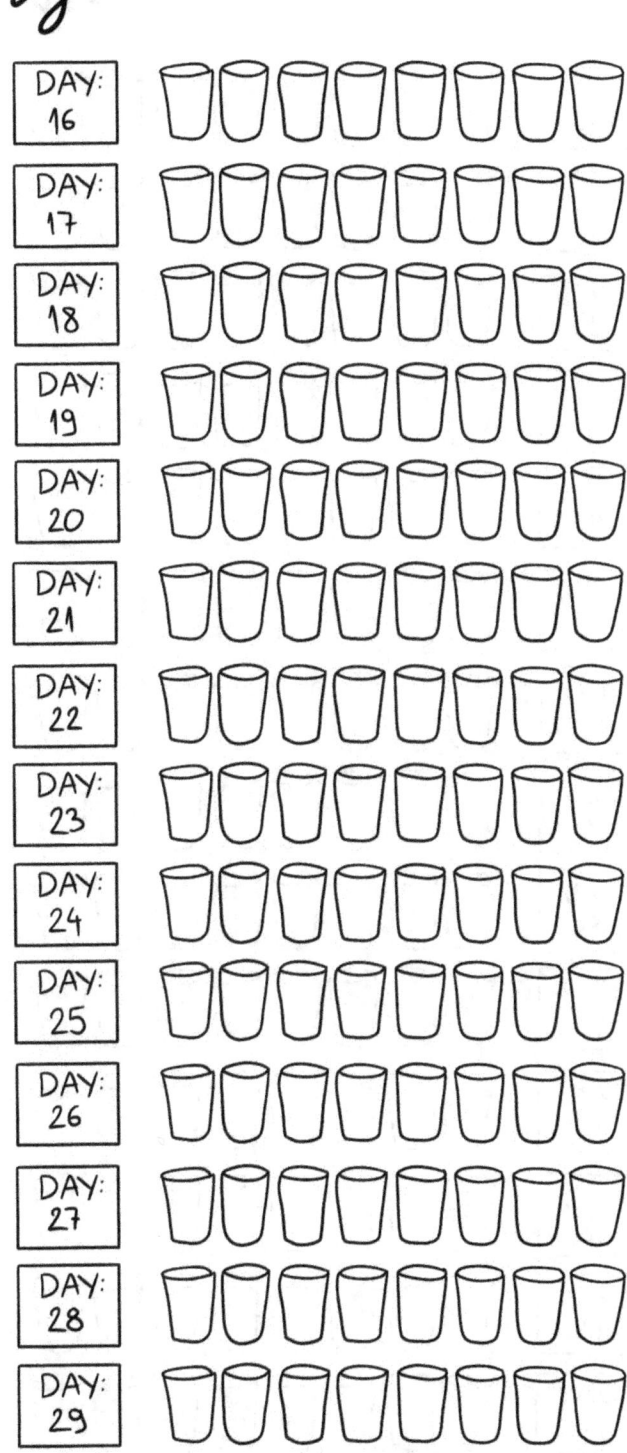

30 DAY
WATER
challenge

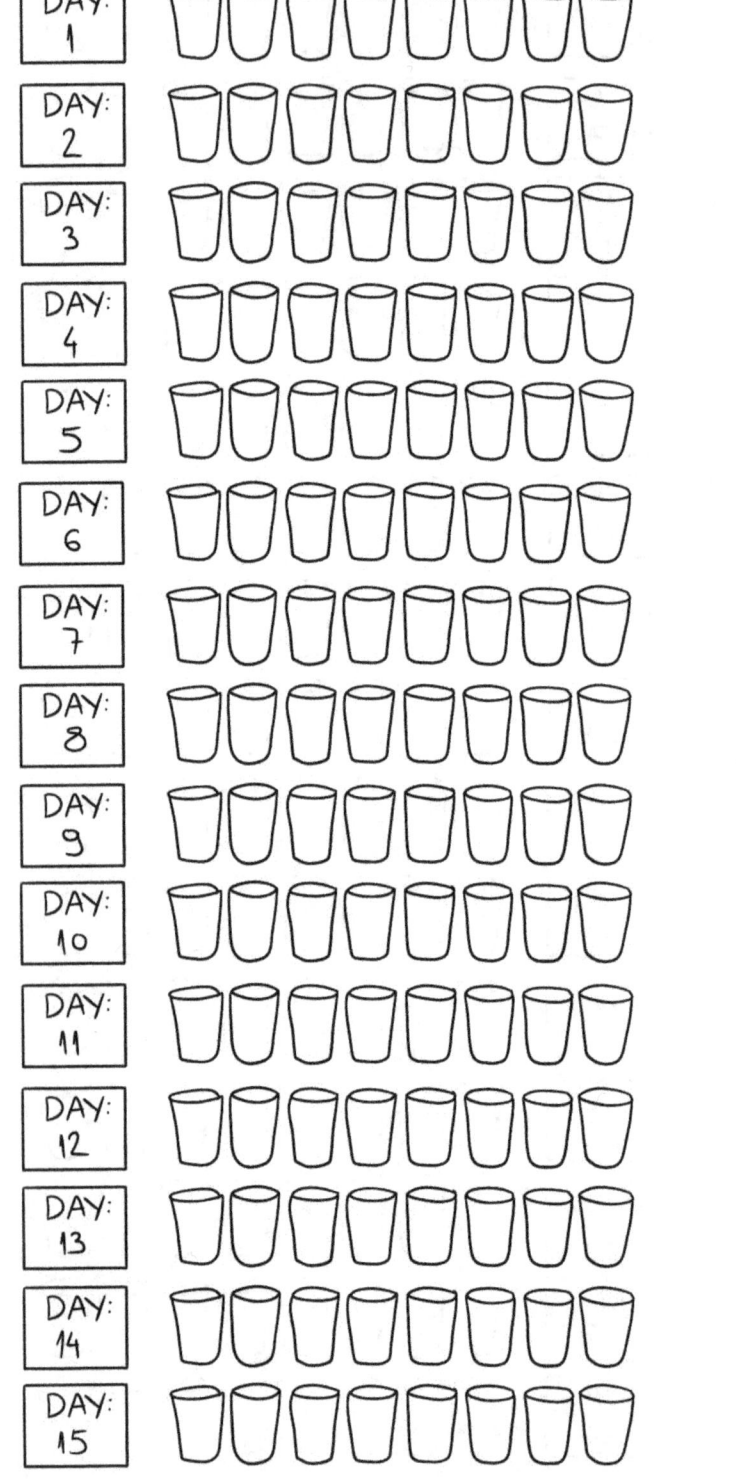

DAY: 1									DAY: 16								
DAY: 2									DAY: 17								
DAY: 3									DAY: 18								
DAY: 4									DAY: 19								
DAY: 5									DAY: 20								
DAY: 6									DAY: 21								
DAY: 7									DAY: 22								
DAY: 8									DAY: 23								
DAY: 9									DAY: 24								
DAY: 10									DAY: 25								
DAY: 11									DAY: 26								
DAY: 12									DAY: 27								
DAY: 13									DAY: 28								
DAY: 14									DAY: 29								
DAY: 15									DAY: 30								

30 DAY
WATER
challenge

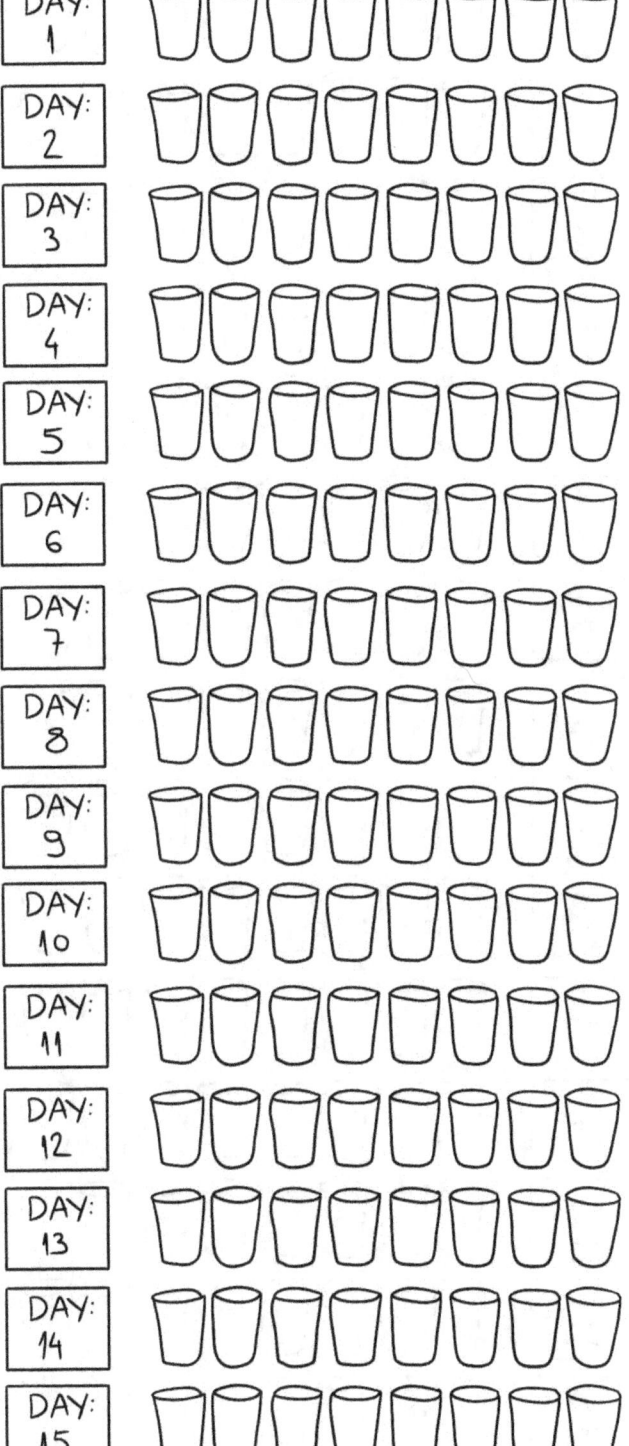

DAY: 1							
DAY: 2							
DAY: 3							
DAY: 4							
DAY: 5							
DAY: 6							
DAY: 7							
DAY: 8							
DAY: 9							
DAY: 10							
DAY: 11							
DAY: 12							
DAY: 13							
DAY: 14							
DAY: 15							

DAY: 16							
DAY: 17							
DAY: 18							
DAY: 19							
DAY: 20							
DAY: 21							
DAY: 22							
DAY: 23							
DAY: 24							
DAY: 25							
DAY: 26							
DAY: 27							
DAY: 28							
DAY: 29							
DAY: 30							

30 DAY
WATER
challenge

DAY: 1

DAY: 2

DAY: 3

DAY: 4

DAY: 5

DAY: 6

DAY: 7

DAY: 8

DAY: 9

DAY: 10

DAY: 11

DAY: 12

DAY: 13

DAY: 14

DAY: 15

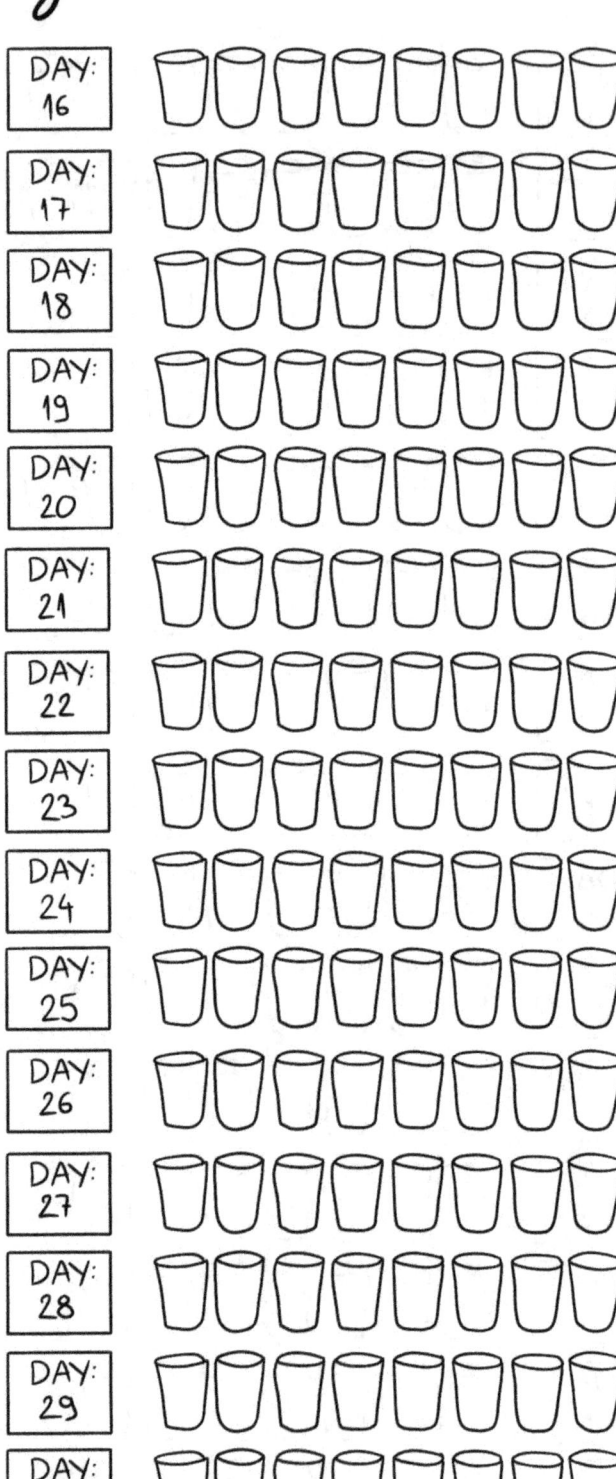

DAY: 16

DAY: 17

DAY: 18

DAY: 19

DAY: 20

DAY: 21

DAY: 22

DAY: 23

DAY: 24

DAY: 25

DAY: 26

DAY: 27

DAY: 28

DAY: 29

DAY: 30

30 DAY
WATER
challenge

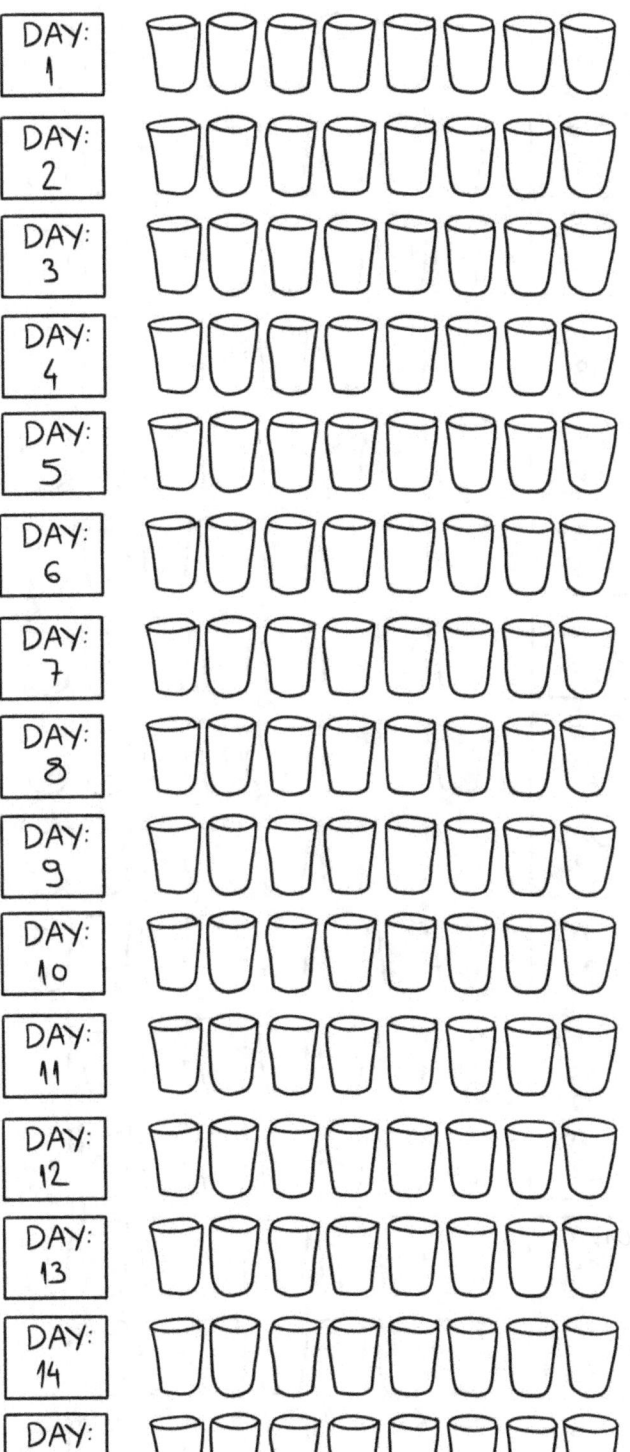

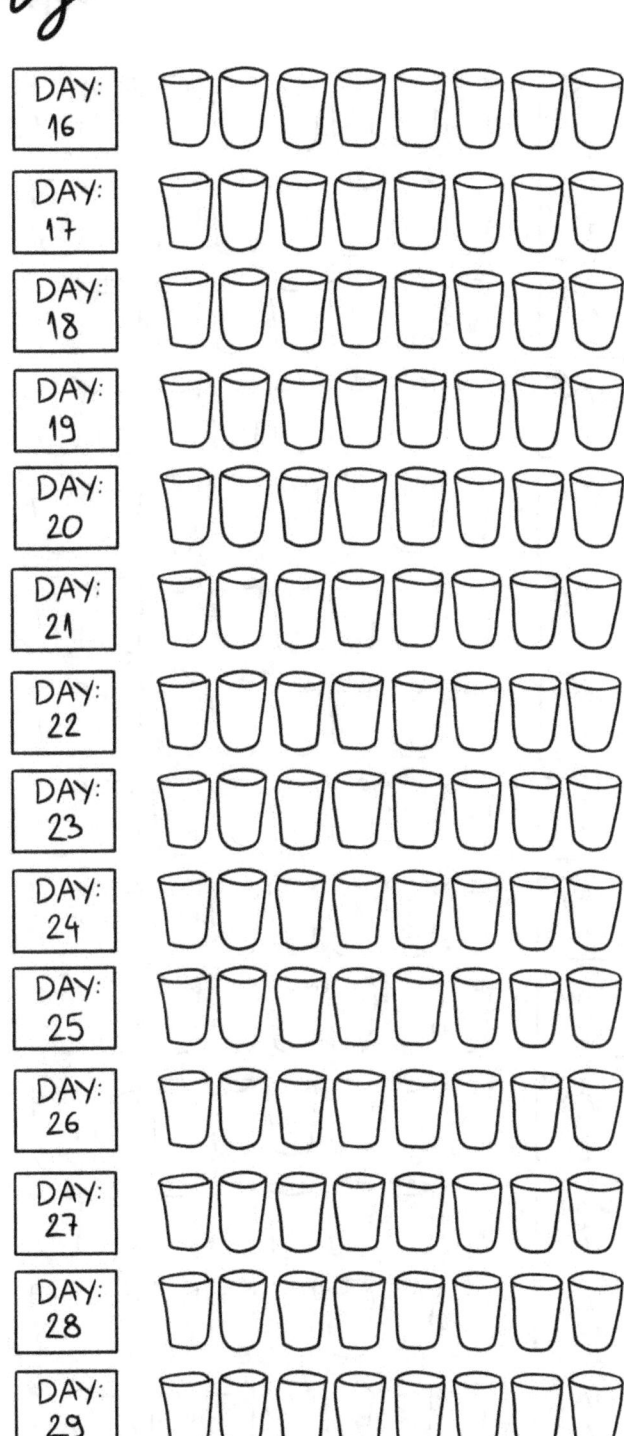

30 DAY
WATER
challenge

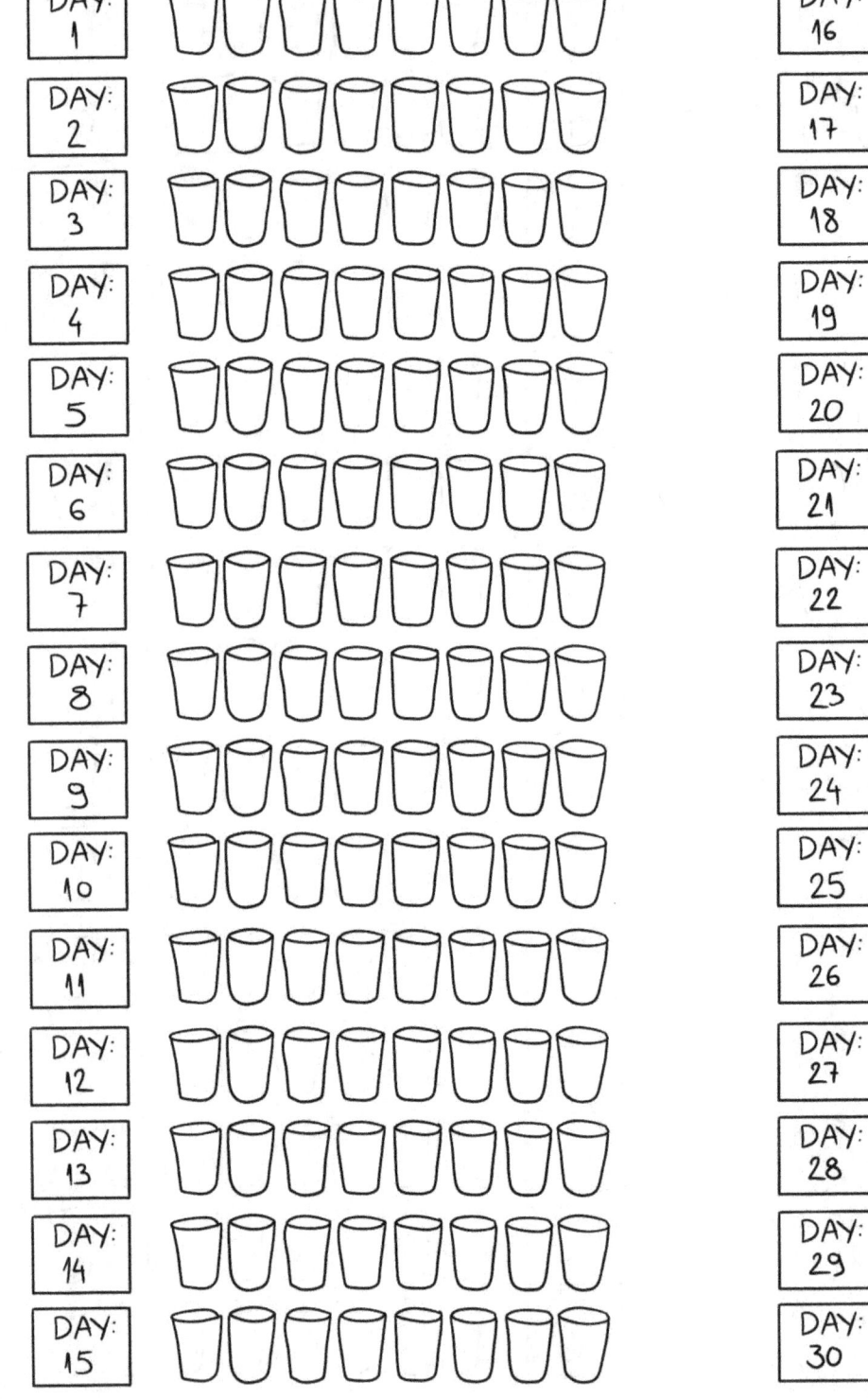

DAY: 1	DAY: 16
DAY: 2	DAY: 17
DAY: 3	DAY: 18
DAY: 4	DAY: 19
DAY: 5	DAY: 20
DAY: 6	DAY: 21
DAY: 7	DAY: 22
DAY: 8	DAY: 23
DAY: 9	DAY: 24
DAY: 10	DAY: 25
DAY: 11	DAY: 26
DAY: 12	DAY: 27
DAY: 13	DAY: 28
DAY: 14	DAY: 29
DAY: 15	DAY: 30

30 DAY
WATER
challenge

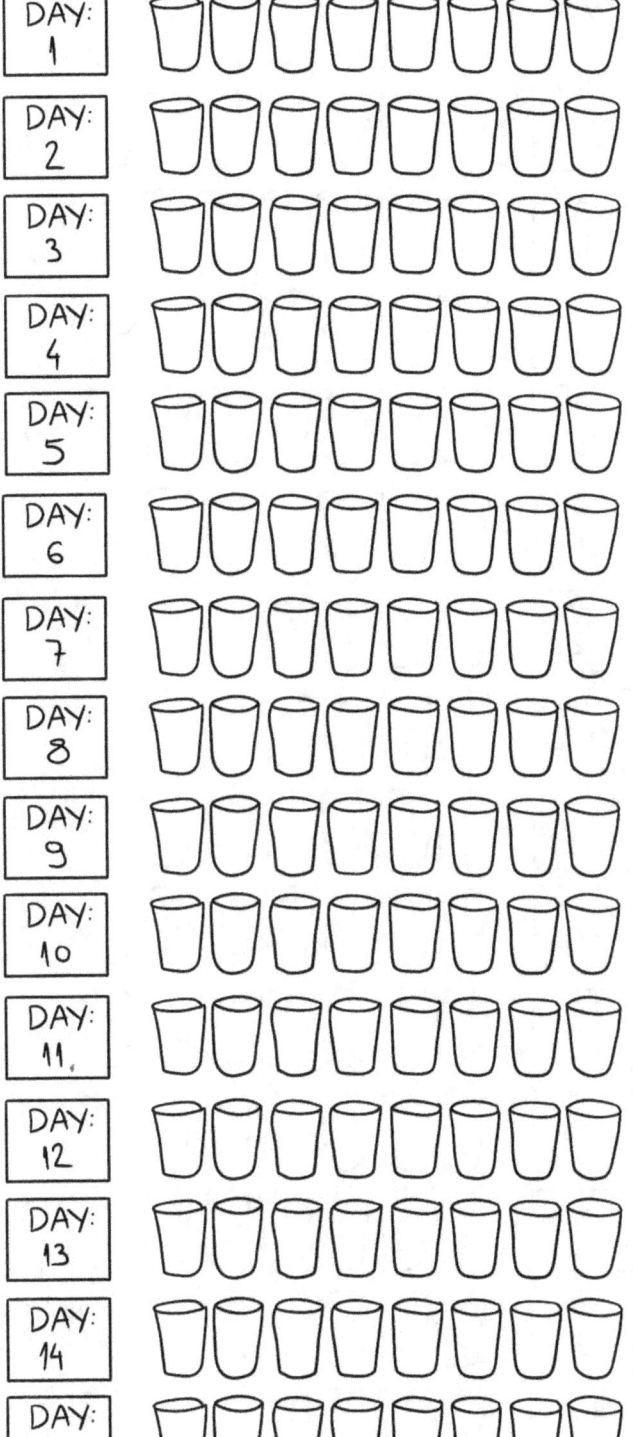

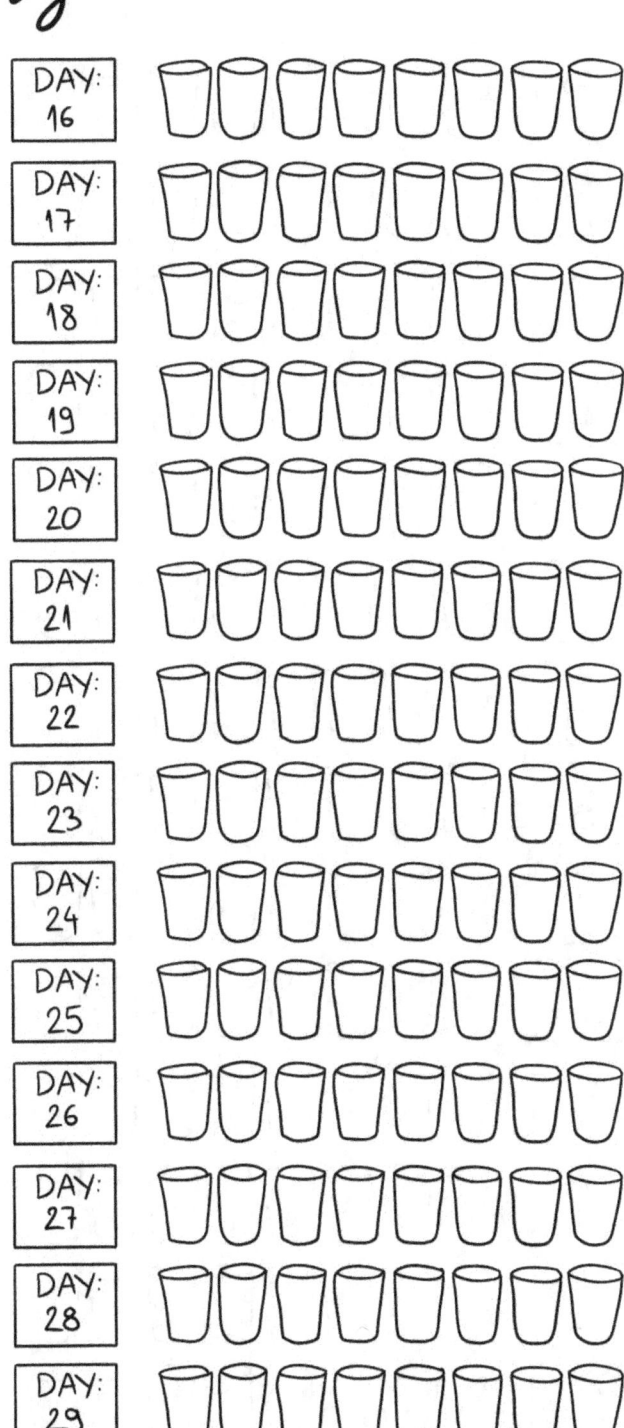

30 DAY
WATER
challenge

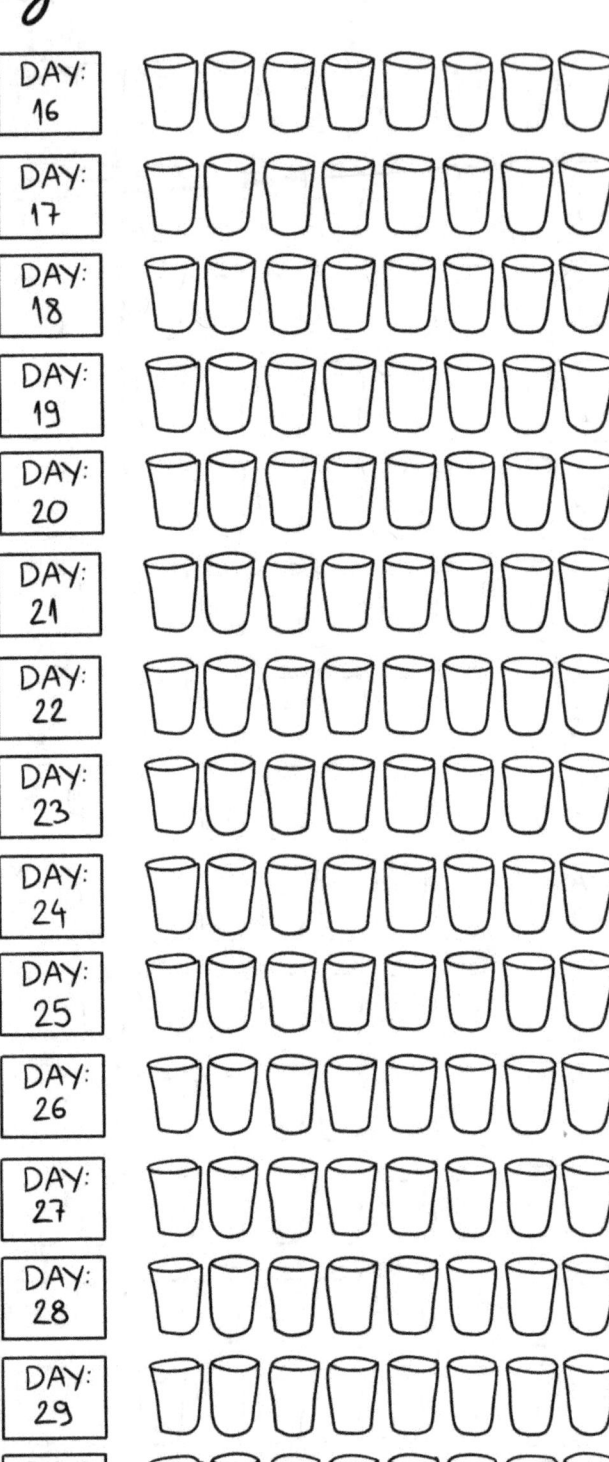

DAY: 1	🥛🥛🥛🥛🥛🥛🥛🥛
DAY: 2	🥛🥛🥛🥛🥛🥛🥛🥛
DAY: 3	🥛🥛🥛🥛🥛🥛🥛🥛
DAY: 4	🥛🥛🥛🥛🥛🥛🥛🥛
DAY: 5	🥛🥛🥛🥛🥛🥛🥛🥛
DAY: 6	🥛🥛🥛🥛🥛🥛🥛🥛
DAY: 7	🥛🥛🥛🥛🥛🥛🥛🥛
DAY: 8	🥛🥛🥛🥛🥛🥛🥛🥛
DAY: 9	🥛🥛🥛🥛🥛🥛🥛🥛
DAY: 10	🥛🥛🥛🥛🥛🥛🥛🥛
DAY: 11	🥛🥛🥛🥛🥛🥛🥛🥛
DAY: 12	🥛🥛🥛🥛🥛🥛🥛🥛
DAY: 13	🥛🥛🥛🥛🥛🥛🥛🥛
DAY: 14	🥛🥛🥛🥛🥛🥛🥛🥛
DAY: 15	🥛🥛🥛🥛🥛🥛🥛🥛

DAY: 16	🥛🥛🥛🥛🥛🥛🥛🥛
DAY: 17	🥛🥛🥛🥛🥛🥛🥛🥛
DAY: 18	🥛🥛🥛🥛🥛🥛🥛🥛
DAY: 19	🥛🥛🥛🥛🥛🥛🥛🥛
DAY: 20	🥛🥛🥛🥛🥛🥛🥛🥛
DAY: 21	🥛🥛🥛🥛🥛🥛🥛🥛
DAY: 22	🥛🥛🥛🥛🥛🥛🥛🥛
DAY: 23	🥛🥛🥛🥛🥛🥛🥛🥛
DAY: 24	🥛🥛🥛🥛🥛🥛🥛🥛
DAY: 25	🥛🥛🥛🥛🥛🥛🥛🥛
DAY: 26	🥛🥛🥛🥛🥛🥛🥛🥛
DAY: 27	🥛🥛🥛🥛🥛🥛🥛🥛
DAY: 28	🥛🥛🥛🥛🥛🥛🥛🥛
DAY: 29	🥛🥛🥛🥛🥛🥛🥛🥛
DAY: 30	🥛🥛🥛🥛🥛🥛🥛🥛

30 DAY
WATER
challenge

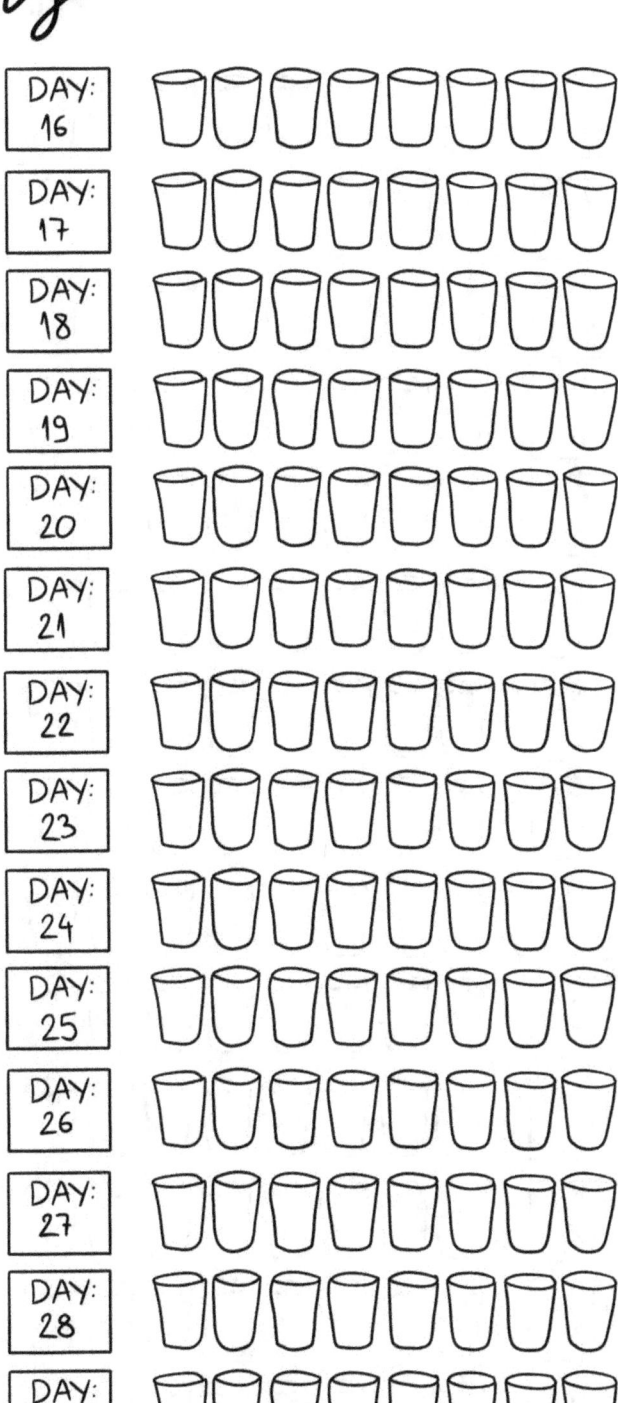

| DAY: 1 |
| DAY: 2 |
| DAY: 3 |
| DAY: 4 |
| DAY: 5 |
| DAY: 6 |
| DAY: 7 |
| DAY: 8 |
| DAY: 9 |
| DAY: 10 |
| DAY: 11 |
| DAY: 12 |
| DAY: 13 |
| DAY: 14 |
| DAY: 15 |

| DAY: 16 |
| DAY: 17 |
| DAY: 18 |
| DAY: 19 |
| DAY: 20 |
| DAY: 21 |
| DAY: 22 |
| DAY: 23 |
| DAY: 24 |
| DAY: 25 |
| DAY: 26 |
| DAY: 27 |
| DAY: 28 |
| DAY: 29 |
| DAY: 30 |

30 DAY
WATER
challenge

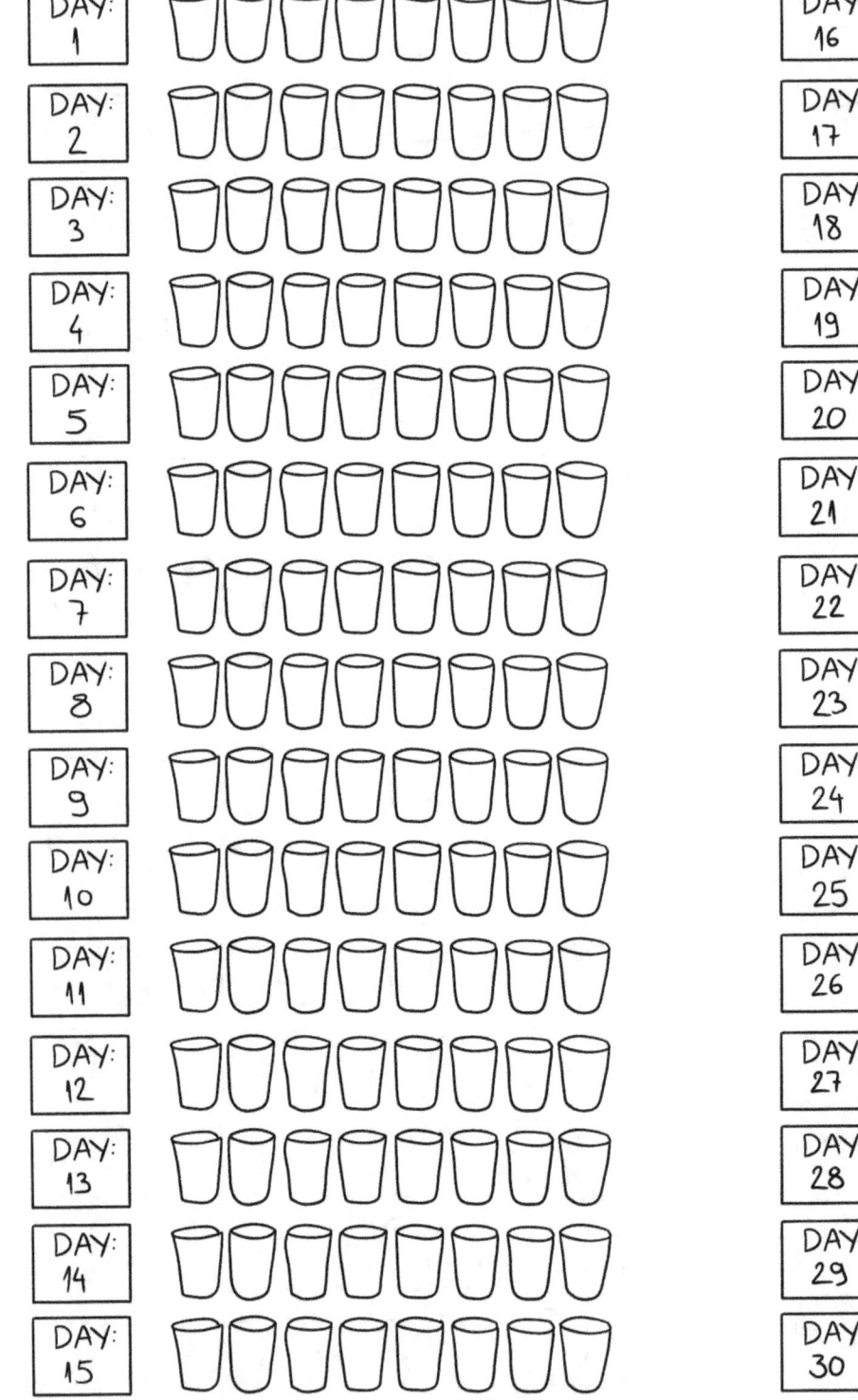

DAY: 1		DAY: 16	
DAY: 2		DAY: 17	
DAY: 3		DAY: 18	
DAY: 4		DAY: 19	
DAY: 5		DAY: 20	
DAY: 6		DAY: 21	
DAY: 7		DAY: 22	
DAY: 8		DAY: 23	
DAY: 9		DAY: 24	
DAY: 10		DAY: 25	
DAY: 11		DAY: 26	
DAY: 12		DAY: 27	
DAY: 13		DAY: 28	
DAY: 14		DAY: 29	
DAY: 15		DAY: 30	

30 DAY
WATER
challenge

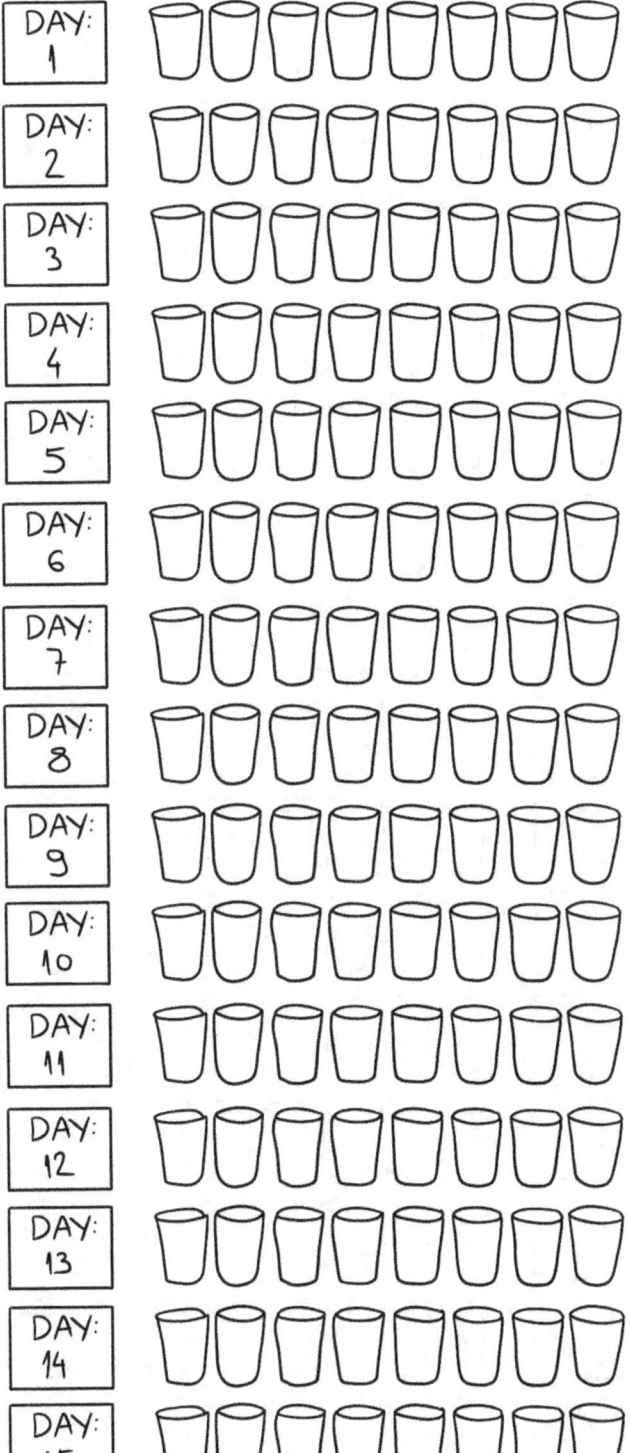

| DAY: 16 |
| DAY: 17 |
| DAY: 18 |
| DAY: 19 |
| DAY: 20 |
| DAY: 21 |
| DAY: 22 |
| DAY: 23 |
| DAY: 24 |
| DAY: 25 |
| DAY: 26 |
| DAY: 27 |
| DAY: 28 |
| DAY: 29 |
| DAY: 30 |

30 DAY
WATER
challenge

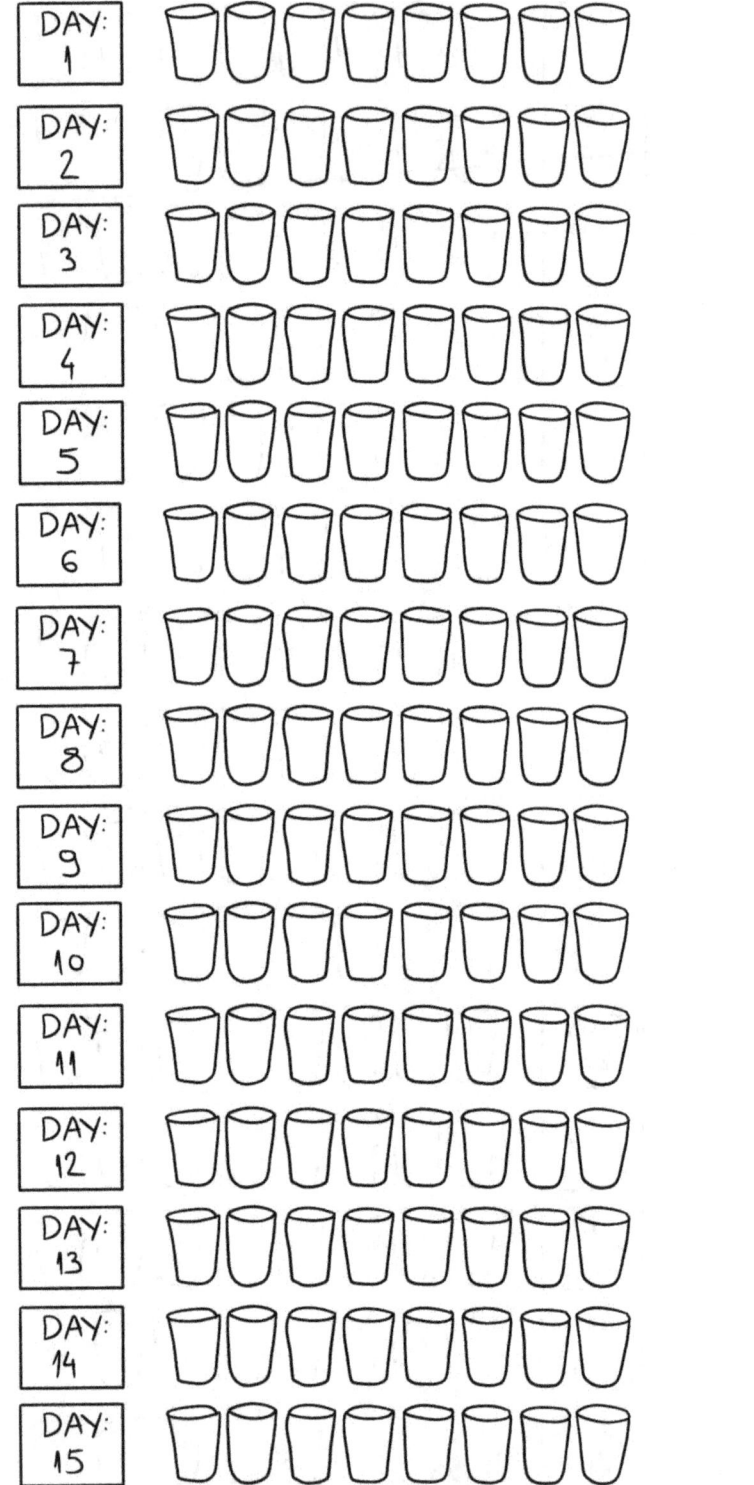
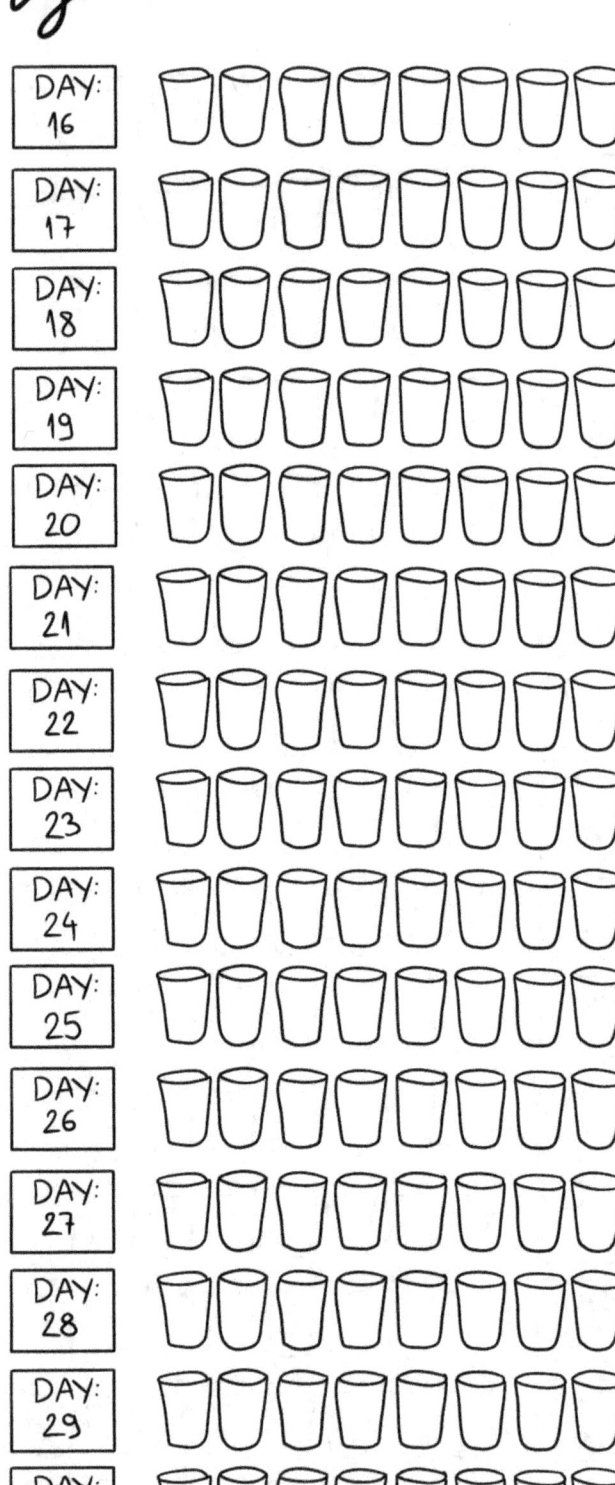

DAY: 1

DAY: 2

DAY: 3

DAY: 4

DAY: 5

DAY: 6

DAY: 7

DAY: 8

DAY: 9

DAY: 10

DAY: 11

DAY: 12

DAY: 13

DAY: 14

DAY: 15

DAY: 16

DAY: 17

DAY: 18

DAY: 19

DAY: 20

DAY: 21

DAY: 22

DAY: 23

DAY: 24

DAY: 25

DAY: 26

DAY: 27

DAY: 28

DAY: 29

DAY: 30

30 DAY
WATER
challenge

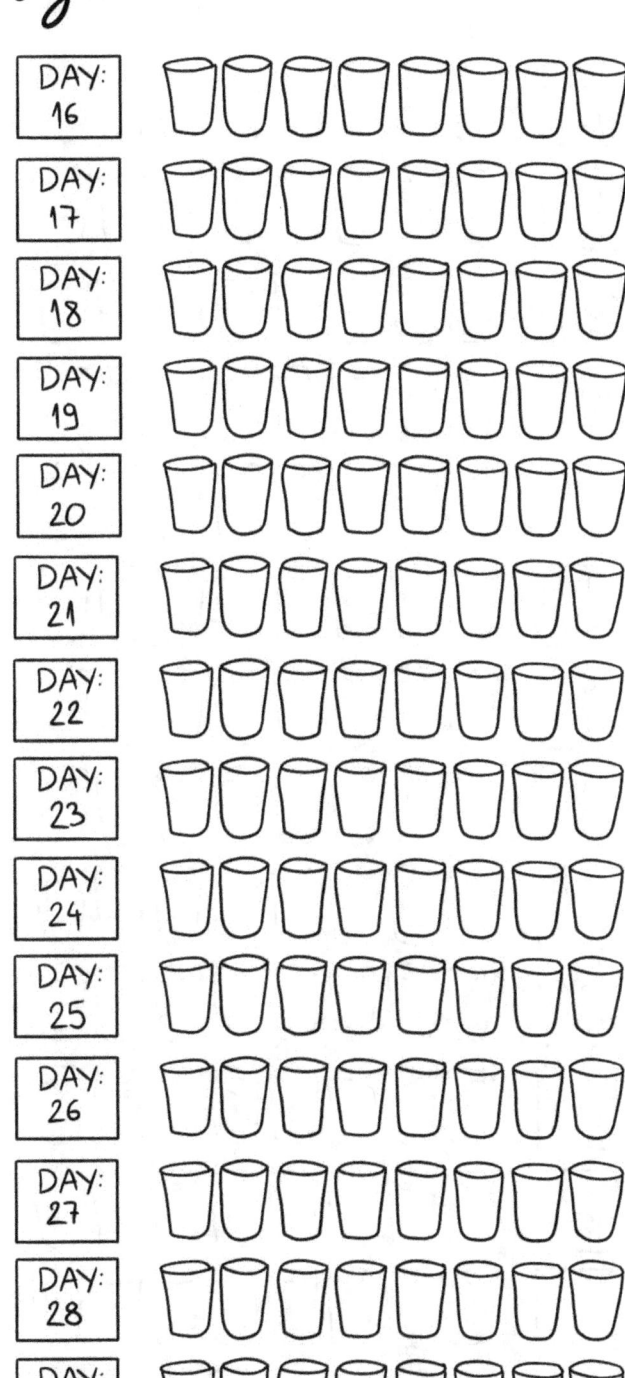

DAY: 1								
DAY: 2								
DAY: 3								
DAY: 4								
DAY: 5								
DAY: 6								
DAY: 7								
DAY: 8								
DAY: 9								
DAY: 10								
DAY: 11								
DAY: 12								
DAY: 13								
DAY: 14								
DAY: 15								

DAY: 16								
DAY: 17								
DAY: 18								
DAY: 19								
DAY: 20								
DAY: 21								
DAY: 22								
DAY: 23								
DAY: 24								
DAY: 25								
DAY: 26								
DAY: 27								
DAY: 28								
DAY: 29								
DAY: 30								

30 DAY
WATER
challenge

DAY: 1								
DAY: 2								
DAY: 3								
DAY: 4								
DAY: 5								
DAY: 6								
DAY: 7								
DAY: 8								
DAY: 9								
DAY: 10								
DAY: 11								
DAY: 12								
DAY: 13								
DAY: 14								
DAY: 15								

DAY: 16								
DAY: 17								
DAY: 18								
DAY: 19								
DAY: 20								
DAY: 21								
DAY: 22								
DAY: 23								
DAY: 24								
DAY: 25								
DAY: 26								
DAY: 27								
DAY: 28								
DAY: 29								
DAY: 30								

30 DAY
WATER
challenge

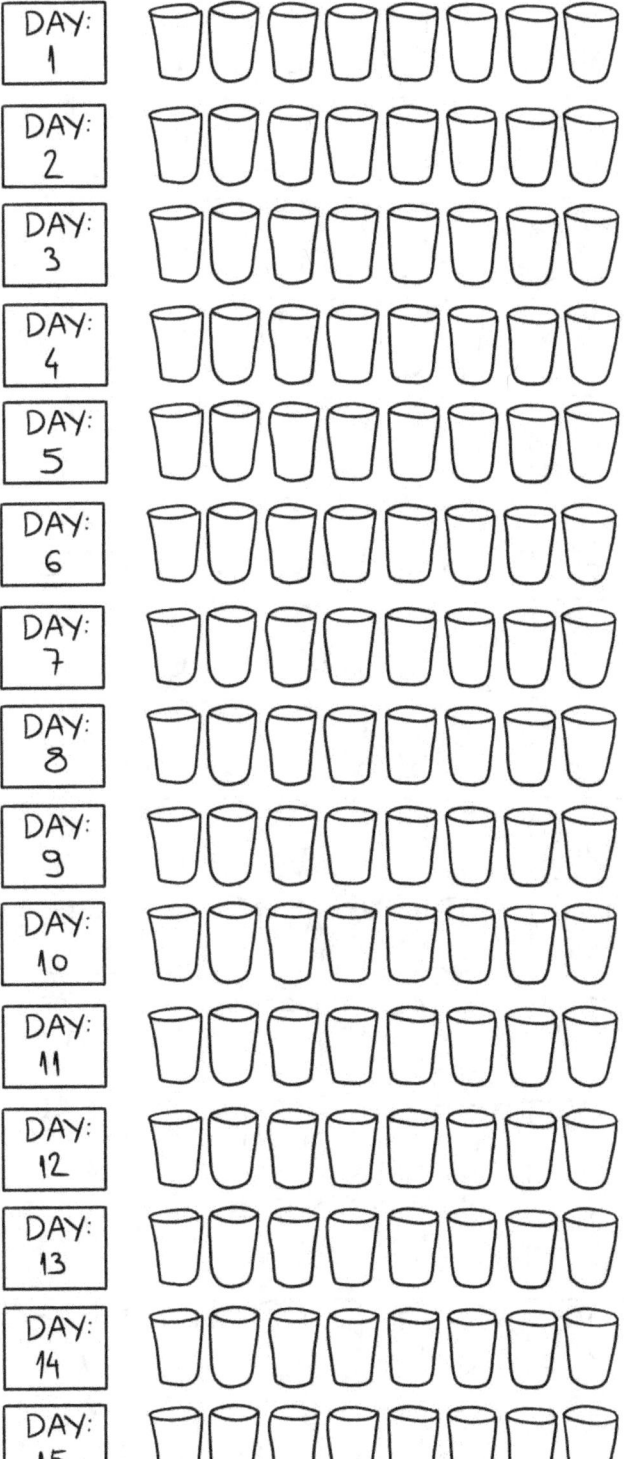

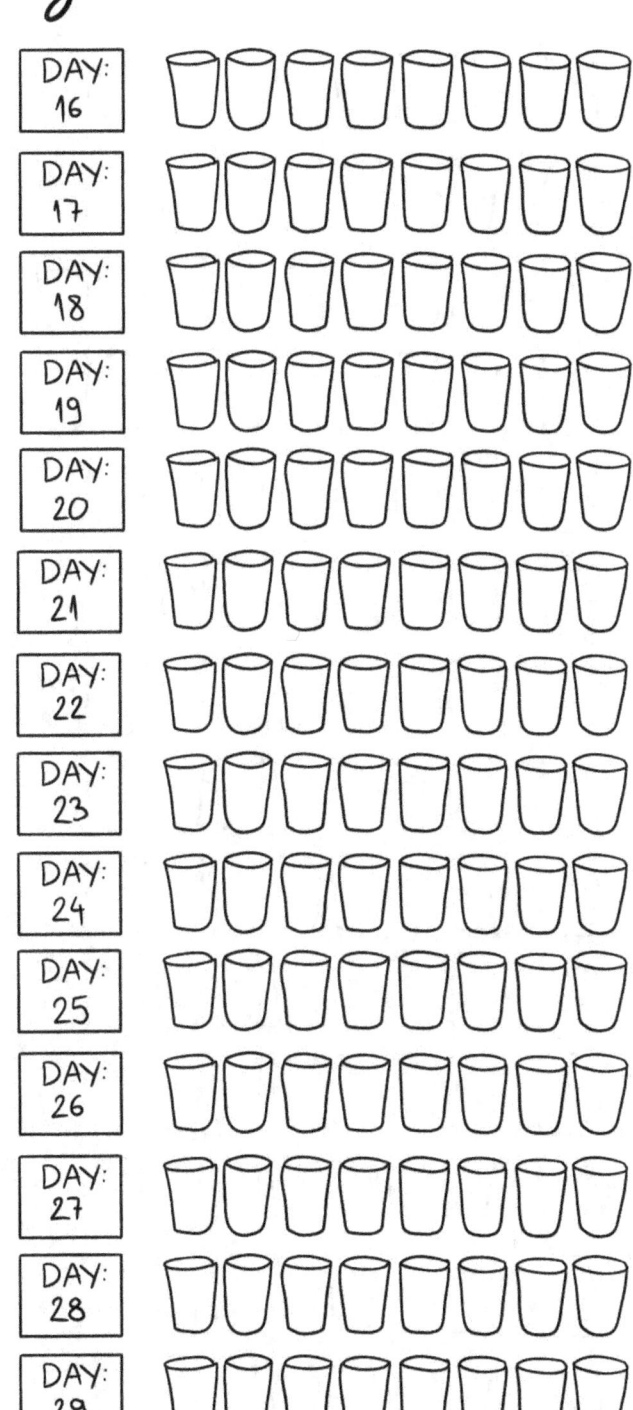

30 DAY
WATER
challenge

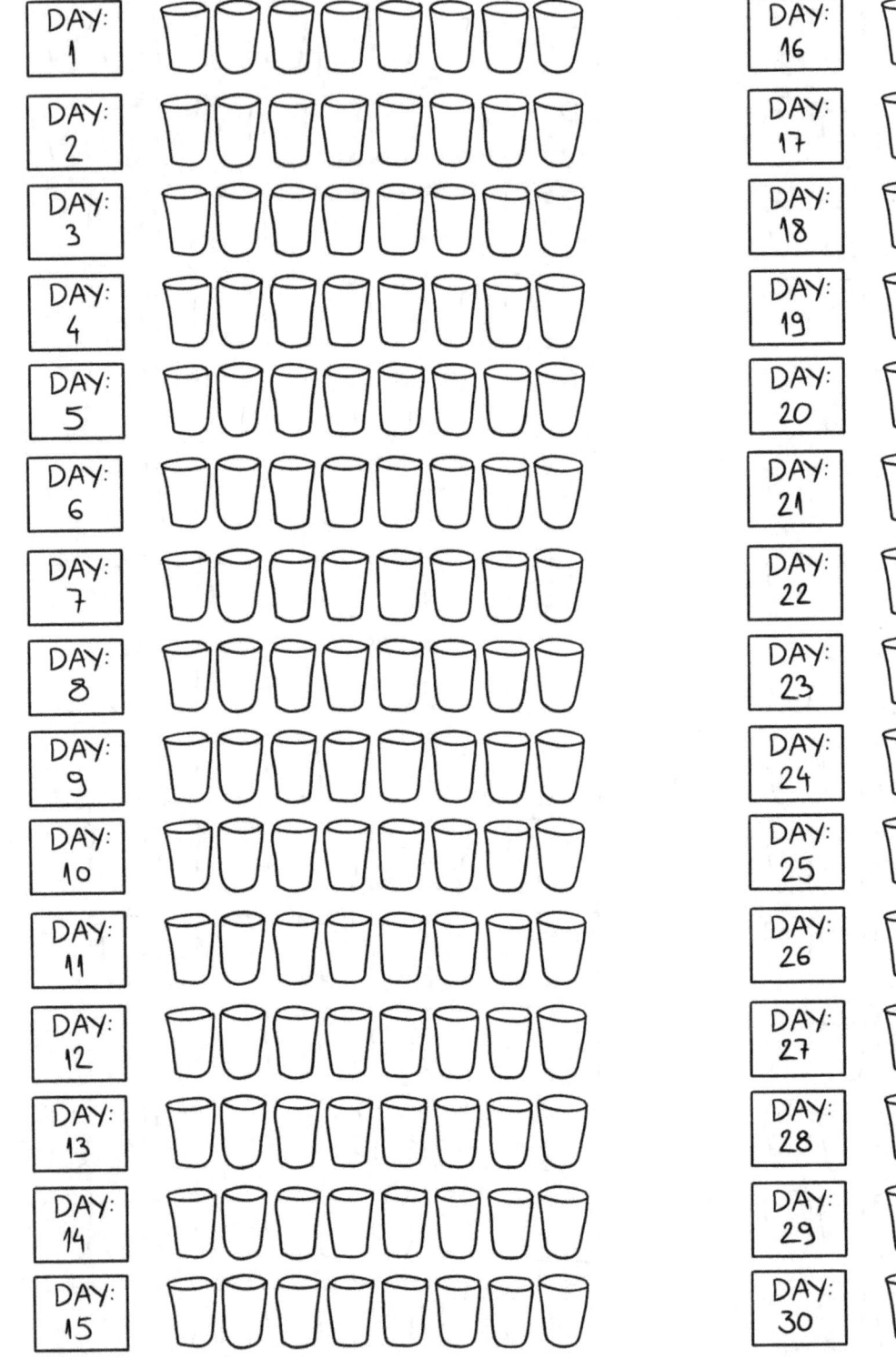

DAY: 1								
DAY: 2								
DAY: 3								
DAY: 4								
DAY: 5								
DAY: 6								
DAY: 7								
DAY: 8								
DAY: 9								
DAY: 10								
DAY: 11								
DAY: 12								
DAY: 13								
DAY: 14								
DAY: 15								

DAY: 16								
DAY: 17								
DAY: 18								
DAY: 19								
DAY: 20								
DAY: 21								
DAY: 22								
DAY: 23								
DAY: 24								
DAY: 25								
DAY: 26								
DAY: 27								
DAY: 28								
DAY: 29								
DAY: 30								

30 DAY
WATER
challenge

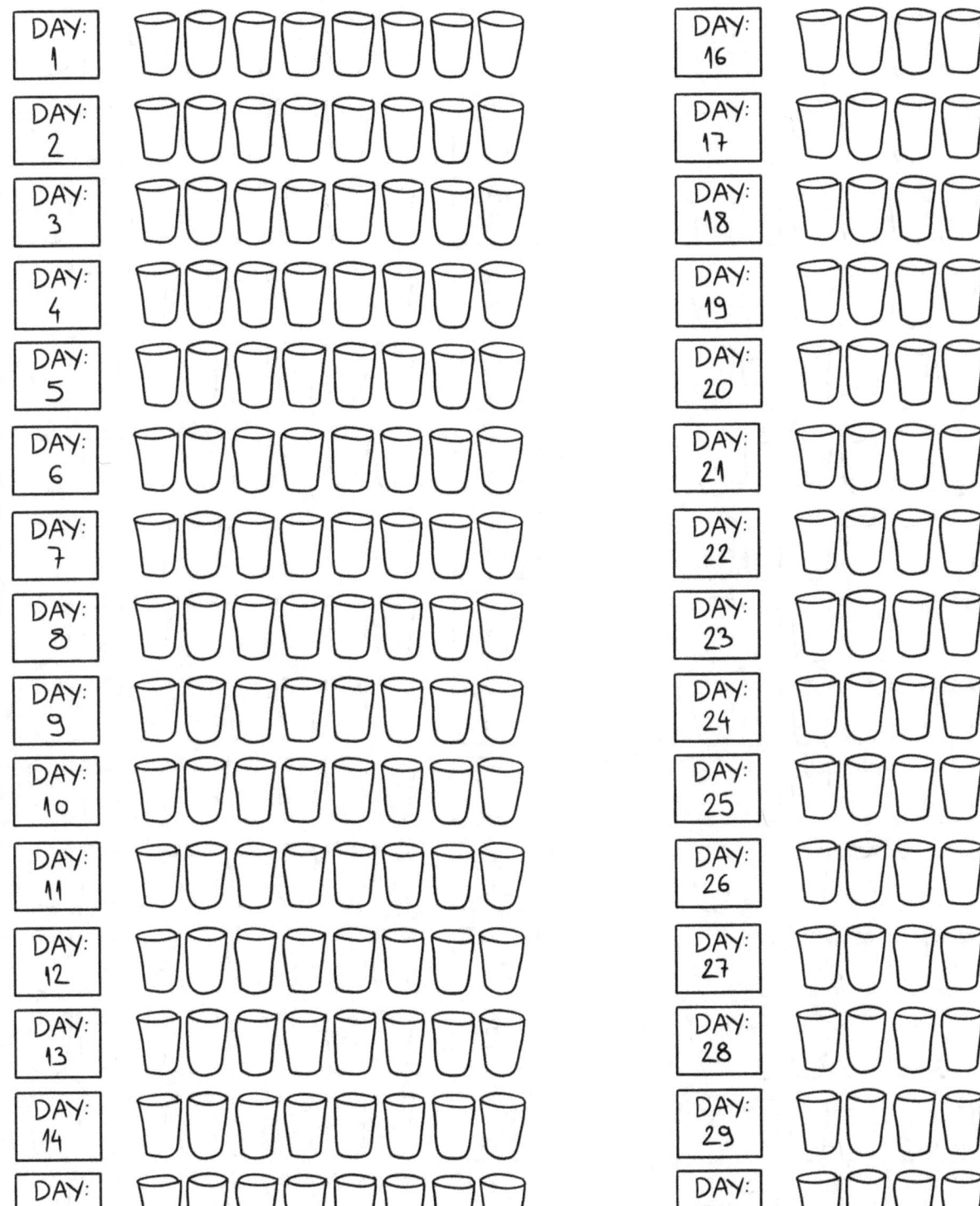

DAY: 1

DAY: 2

DAY: 3

DAY: 4

DAY: 5

DAY: 6

DAY: 7

DAY: 8

DAY: 9

DAY: 10

DAY: 11

DAY: 12

DAY: 13

DAY: 14

DAY: 15

DAY: 16

DAY: 17

DAY: 18

DAY: 19

DAY: 20

DAY: 21

DAY: 22

DAY: 23

DAY: 24

DAY: 25

DAY: 26

DAY: 27

DAY: 28

DAY: 29

DAY: 30

30 DAY
WATER
challenge

DAY: 1	⬜⬜⬜⬜⬜⬜⬜⬜	DAY: 16	⬜⬜⬜⬜⬜⬜⬜⬜
DAY: 2	⬜⬜⬜⬜⬜⬜⬜⬜	DAY: 17	⬜⬜⬜⬜⬜⬜⬜⬜
DAY: 3	⬜⬜⬜⬜⬜⬜⬜⬜	DAY: 18	⬜⬜⬜⬜⬜⬜⬜⬜
DAY: 4	⬜⬜⬜⬜⬜⬜⬜⬜	DAY: 19	⬜⬜⬜⬜⬜⬜⬜⬜
DAY: 5	⬜⬜⬜⬜⬜⬜⬜⬜	DAY: 20	⬜⬜⬜⬜⬜⬜⬜⬜
DAY: 6	⬜⬜⬜⬜⬜⬜⬜⬜	DAY: 21	⬜⬜⬜⬜⬜⬜⬜⬜
DAY: 7	⬜⬜⬜⬜⬜⬜⬜⬜	DAY: 22	⬜⬜⬜⬜⬜⬜⬜⬜
DAY: 8	⬜⬜⬜⬜⬜⬜⬜⬜	DAY: 23	⬜⬜⬜⬜⬜⬜⬜⬜
DAY: 9	⬜⬜⬜⬜⬜⬜⬜⬜	DAY: 24	⬜⬜⬜⬜⬜⬜⬜⬜
DAY: 10	⬜⬜⬜⬜⬜⬜⬜⬜	DAY: 25	⬜⬜⬜⬜⬜⬜⬜⬜
DAY: 11	⬜⬜⬜⬜⬜⬜⬜⬜	DAY: 26	⬜⬜⬜⬜⬜⬜⬜⬜
DAY: 12	⬜⬜⬜⬜⬜⬜⬜⬜	DAY: 27	⬜⬜⬜⬜⬜⬜⬜⬜
DAY: 13	⬜⬜⬜⬜⬜⬜⬜⬜	DAY: 28	⬜⬜⬜⬜⬜⬜⬜⬜
DAY: 14	⬜⬜⬜⬜⬜⬜⬜⬜	DAY: 29	⬜⬜⬜⬜⬜⬜⬜⬜
DAY: 15	⬜⬜⬜⬜⬜⬜⬜⬜	DAY: 30	⬜⬜⬜⬜⬜⬜⬜⬜

30 DAY
WATER
challenge

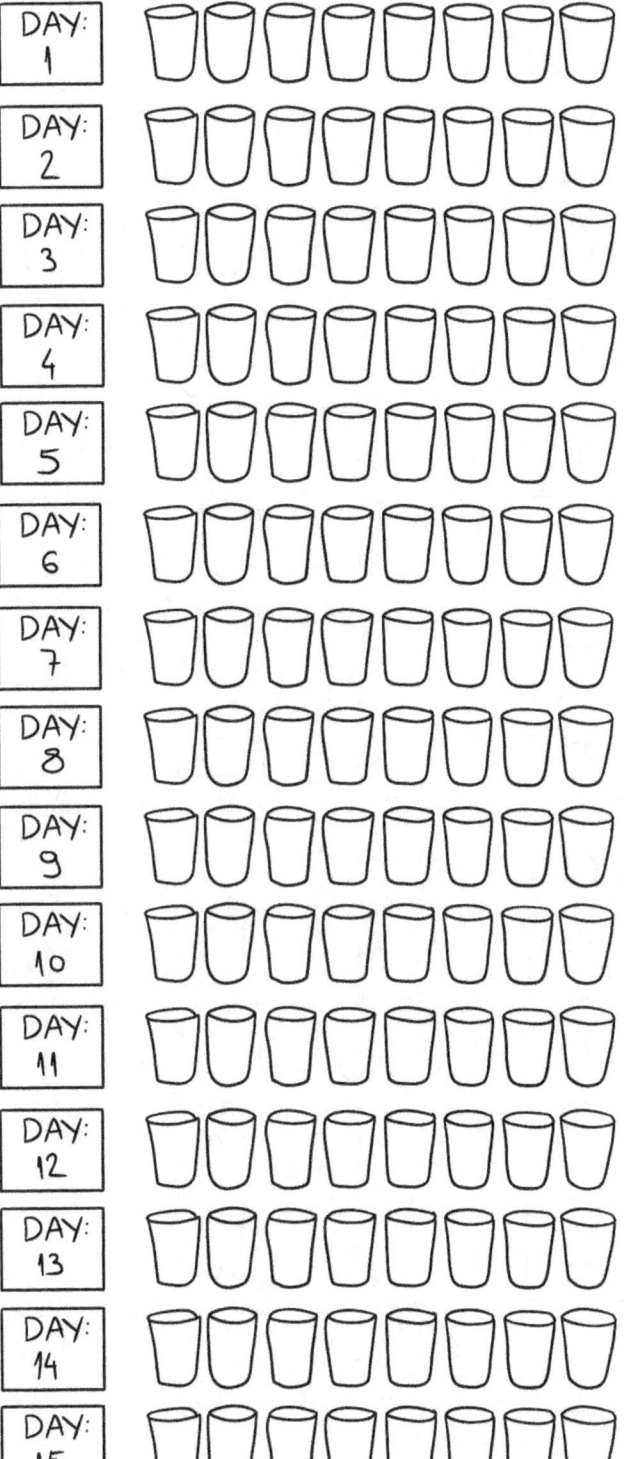

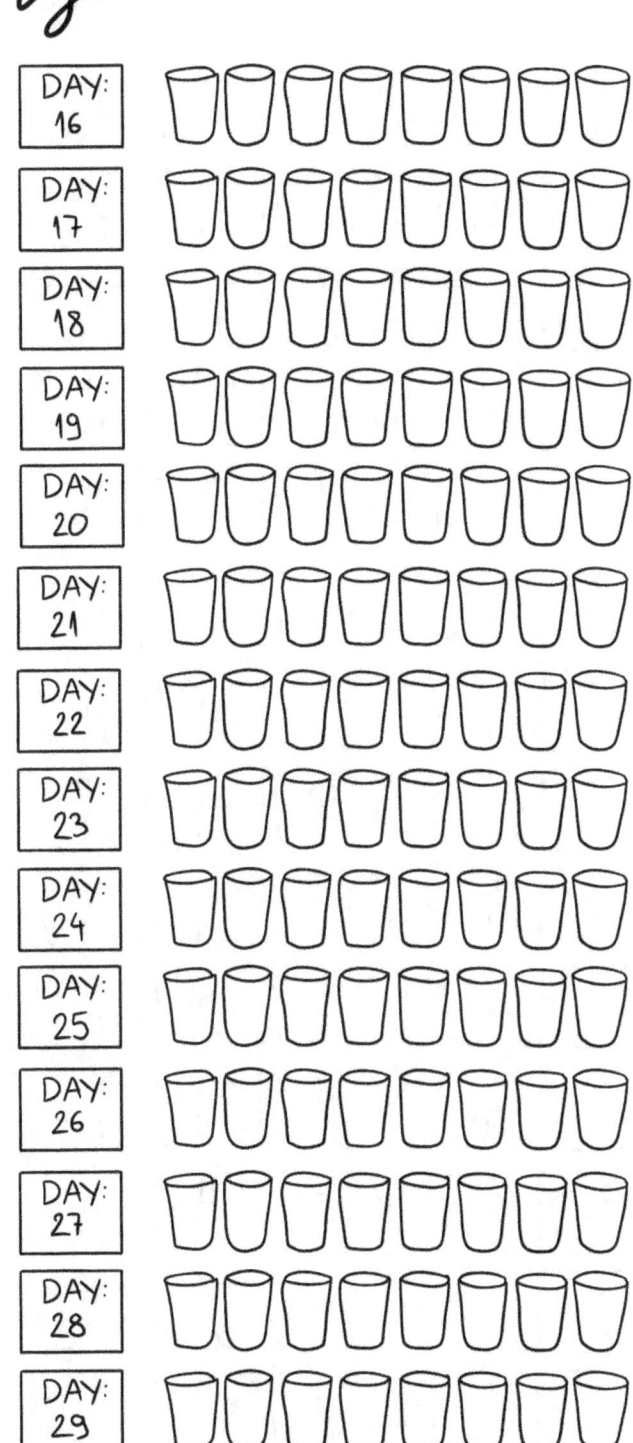

30 DAY
WATER
challenge

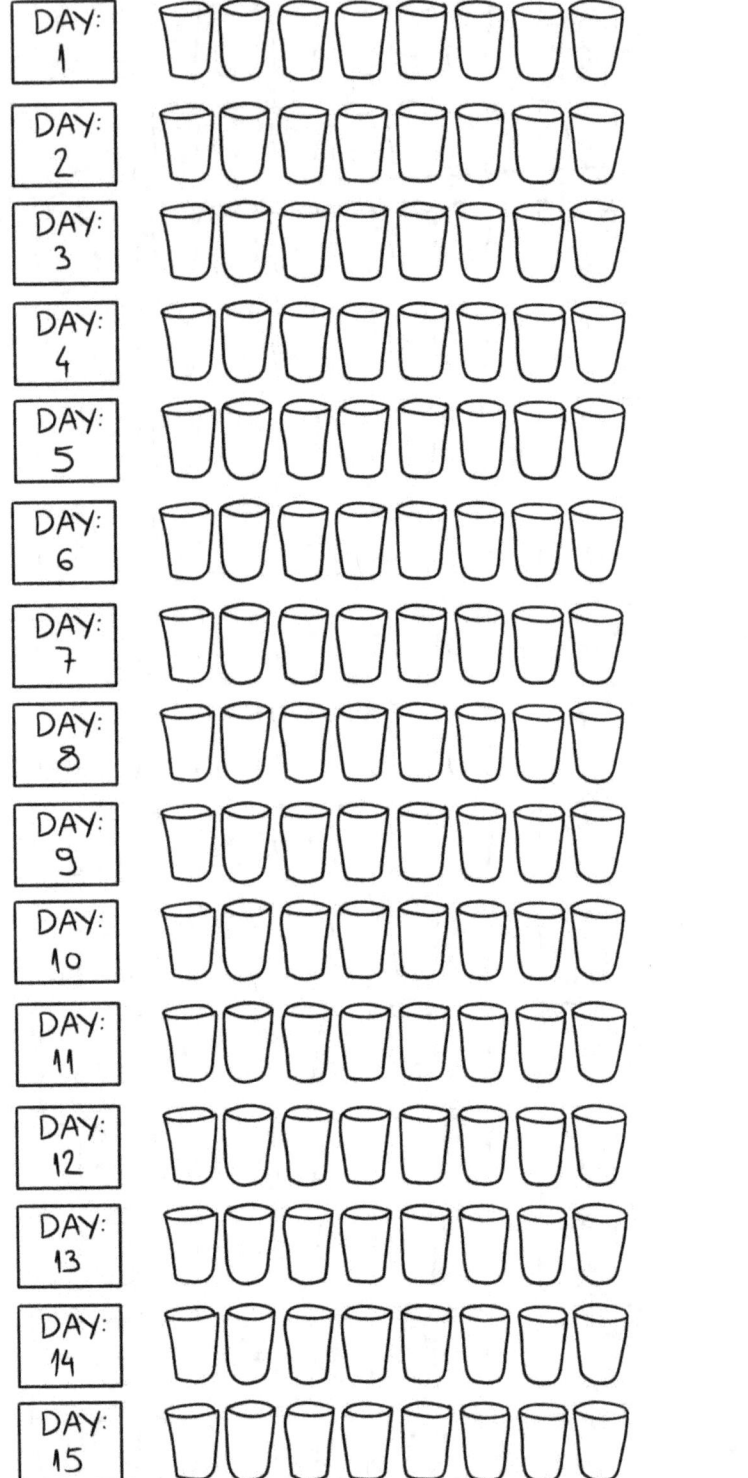

DAY: 1								DAY: 16							
DAY: 2								DAY: 17							
DAY: 3								DAY: 18							
DAY: 4								DAY: 19							
DAY: 5								DAY: 20							
DAY: 6								DAY: 21							
DAY: 7								DAY: 22							
DAY: 8								DAY: 23							
DAY: 9								DAY: 24							
DAY: 10								DAY: 25							
DAY: 11								DAY: 26							
DAY: 12								DAY: 27							
DAY: 13								DAY: 28							
DAY: 14								DAY: 29							
DAY: 15								DAY: 30							

30 DAY WATER challenge

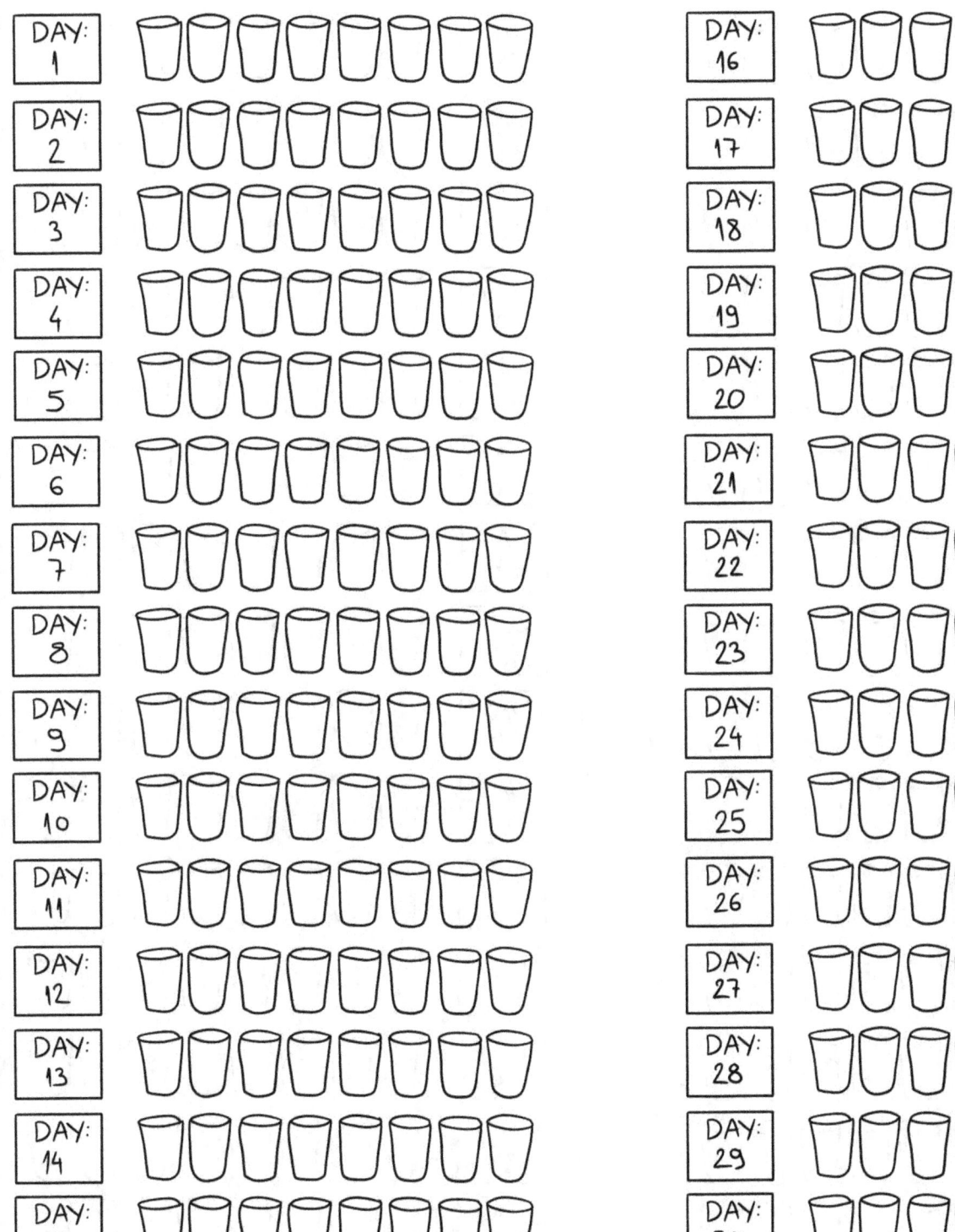

DAY: 1									DAY: 16							
DAY: 2									DAY: 17							
DAY: 3									DAY: 18							
DAY: 4									DAY: 19							
DAY: 5									DAY: 20							
DAY: 6									DAY: 21							
DAY: 7									DAY: 22							
DAY: 8									DAY: 23							
DAY: 9									DAY: 24							
DAY: 10									DAY: 25							
DAY: 11									DAY: 26							
DAY: 12									DAY: 27							
DAY: 13									DAY: 28							
DAY: 14									DAY: 29							
DAY: 15									DAY: 30							

30 DAY WATER challenge

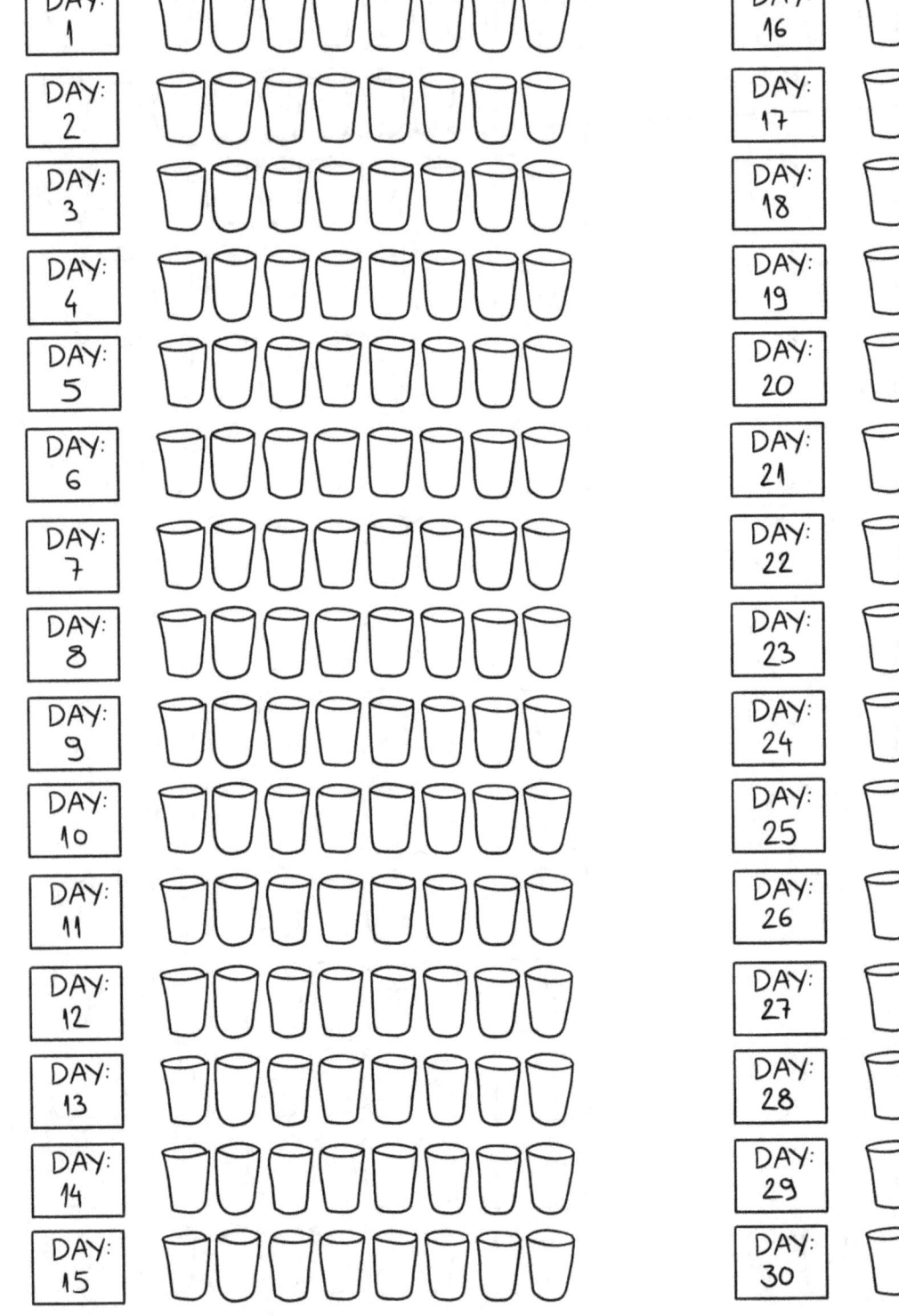

30 DAY
WATER
challenge

DAY: 1	☐☐☐☐☐☐☐☐
DAY: 2	☐☐☐☐☐☐☐☐
DAY: 3	☐☐☐☐☐☐☐☐
DAY: 4	☐☐☐☐☐☐☐☐
DAY: 5	☐☐☐☐☐☐☐☐
DAY: 6	☐☐☐☐☐☐☐☐
DAY: 7	☐☐☐☐☐☐☐☐
DAY: 8	☐☐☐☐☐☐☐☐
DAY: 9	☐☐☐☐☐☐☐☐
DAY: 10	☐☐☐☐☐☐☐☐
DAY: 11	☐☐☐☐☐☐☐☐
DAY: 12	☐☐☐☐☐☐☐☐
DAY: 13	☐☐☐☐☐☐☐☐
DAY: 14	☐☐☐☐☐☐☐☐
DAY: 15	☐☐☐☐☐☐☐☐

DAY: 16	☐☐☐☐☐☐☐☐
DAY: 17	☐☐☐☐☐☐☐☐
DAY: 18	☐☐☐☐☐☐☐☐
DAY: 19	☐☐☐☐☐☐☐☐
DAY: 20	☐☐☐☐☐☐☐☐
DAY: 21	☐☐☐☐☐☐☐☐
DAY: 22	☐☐☐☐☐☐☐☐
DAY: 23	☐☐☐☐☐☐☐☐
DAY: 24	☐☐☐☐☐☐☐☐
DAY: 25	☐☐☐☐☐☐☐☐
DAY: 26	☐☐☐☐☐☐☐☐
DAY: 27	☐☐☐☐☐☐☐☐
DAY: 28	☐☐☐☐☐☐☐☐
DAY: 29	☐☐☐☐☐☐☐☐
DAY: 30	☐☐☐☐☐☐☐☐

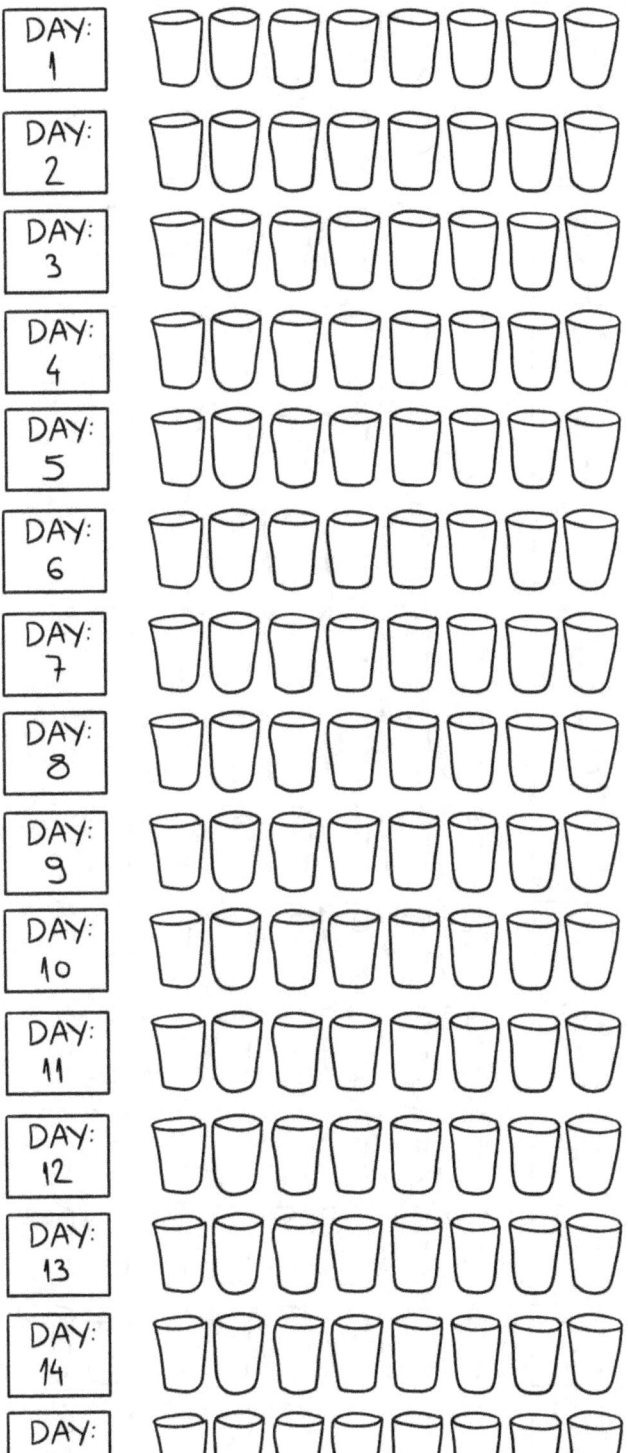

30 DAY
WATER
challenge

DAY: 1	🥛🥛🥛🥛🥛🥛🥛🥛
DAY: 2	🥛🥛🥛🥛🥛🥛🥛🥛
DAY: 3	🥛🥛🥛🥛🥛🥛🥛🥛
DAY: 4	🥛🥛🥛🥛🥛🥛🥛🥛
DAY: 5	🥛🥛🥛🥛🥛🥛🥛🥛
DAY: 6	🥛🥛🥛🥛🥛🥛🥛🥛
DAY: 7	🥛🥛🥛🥛🥛🥛🥛🥛
DAY: 8	🥛🥛🥛🥛🥛🥛🥛🥛
DAY: 9	🥛🥛🥛🥛🥛🥛🥛🥛
DAY: 10	🥛🥛🥛🥛🥛🥛🥛🥛
DAY: 11	🥛🥛🥛🥛🥛🥛🥛🥛
DAY: 12	🥛🥛🥛🥛🥛🥛🥛🥛
DAY: 13	🥛🥛🥛🥛🥛🥛🥛🥛
DAY: 14	🥛🥛🥛🥛🥛🥛🥛🥛
DAY: 15	🥛🥛🥛🥛🥛🥛🥛🥛

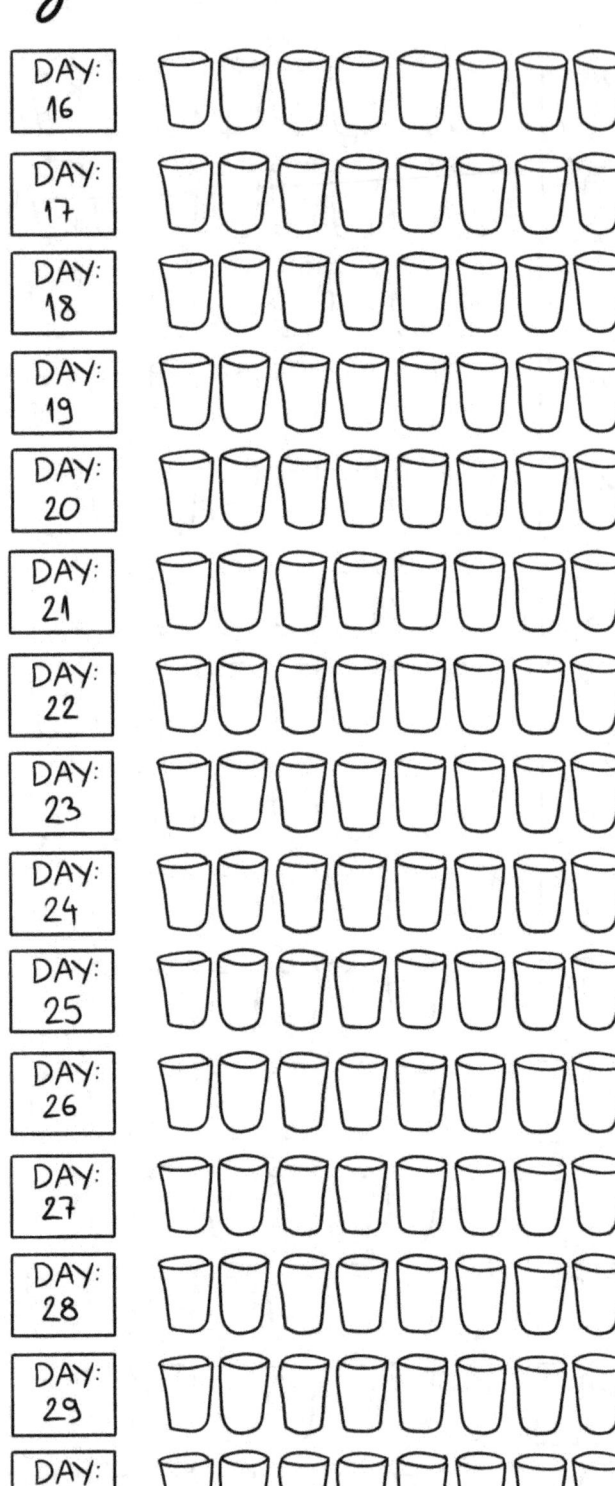

DAY: 16	🥛🥛🥛🥛🥛🥛🥛🥛
DAY: 17	🥛🥛🥛🥛🥛🥛🥛🥛
DAY: 18	🥛🥛🥛🥛🥛🥛🥛🥛
DAY: 19	🥛🥛🥛🥛🥛🥛🥛🥛
DAY: 20	🥛🥛🥛🥛🥛🥛🥛🥛
DAY: 21	🥛🥛🥛🥛🥛🥛🥛🥛
DAY: 22	🥛🥛🥛🥛🥛🥛🥛🥛
DAY: 23	🥛🥛🥛🥛🥛🥛🥛🥛
DAY: 24	🥛🥛🥛🥛🥛🥛🥛🥛
DAY: 25	🥛🥛🥛🥛🥛🥛🥛🥛
DAY: 26	🥛🥛🥛🥛🥛🥛🥛🥛
DAY: 27	🥛🥛🥛🥛🥛🥛🥛🥛
DAY: 28	🥛🥛🥛🥛🥛🥛🥛🥛
DAY: 29	🥛🥛🥛🥛🥛🥛🥛🥛
DAY: 30	🥛🥛🥛🥛🥛🥛🥛🥛

30 DAY
WATER
challenge

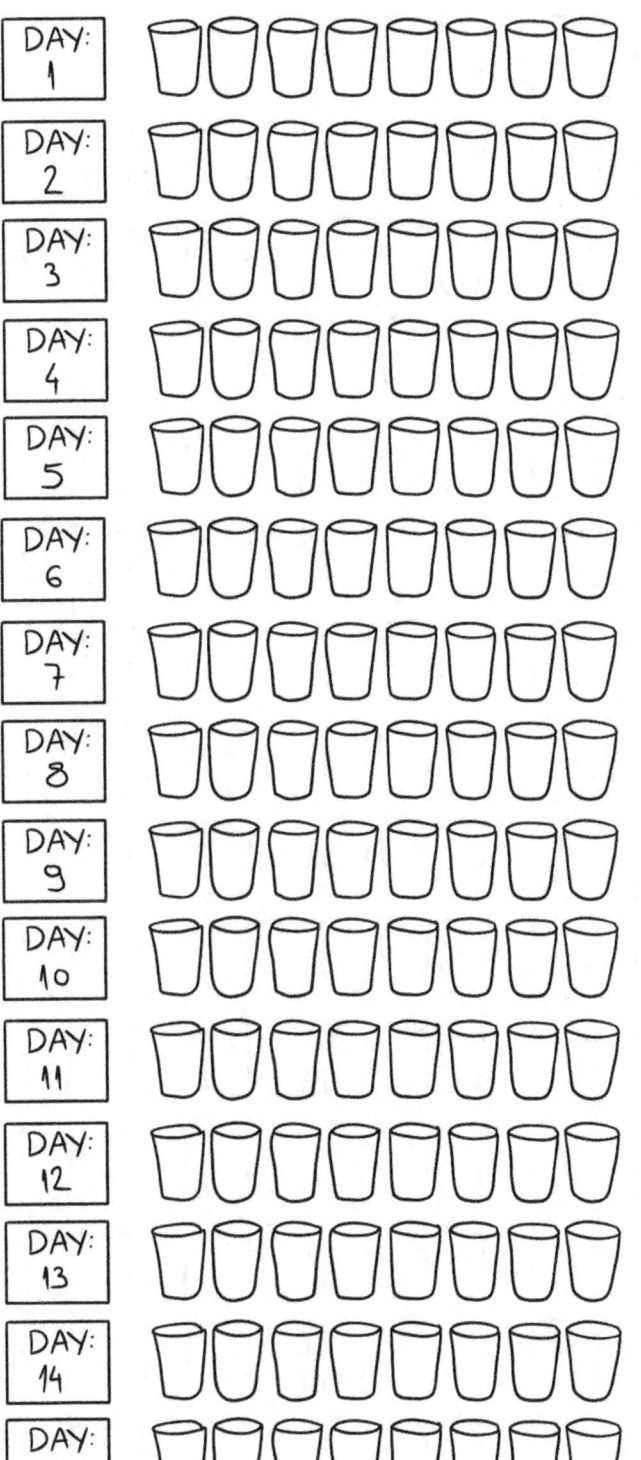

DAY: 1							
DAY: 2							
DAY: 3							
DAY: 4							
DAY: 5							
DAY: 6							
DAY: 7							
DAY: 8							
DAY: 9							
DAY: 10							
DAY: 11							
DAY: 12							
DAY: 13							
DAY: 14							
DAY: 15							

DAY: 16							
DAY: 17							
DAY: 18							
DAY: 19							
DAY: 20							
DAY: 21							
DAY: 22							
DAY: 23							
DAY: 24							
DAY: 25							
DAY: 26							
DAY: 27							
DAY: 28							
DAY: 29							
DAY: 30							

30 DAY WATER challenge

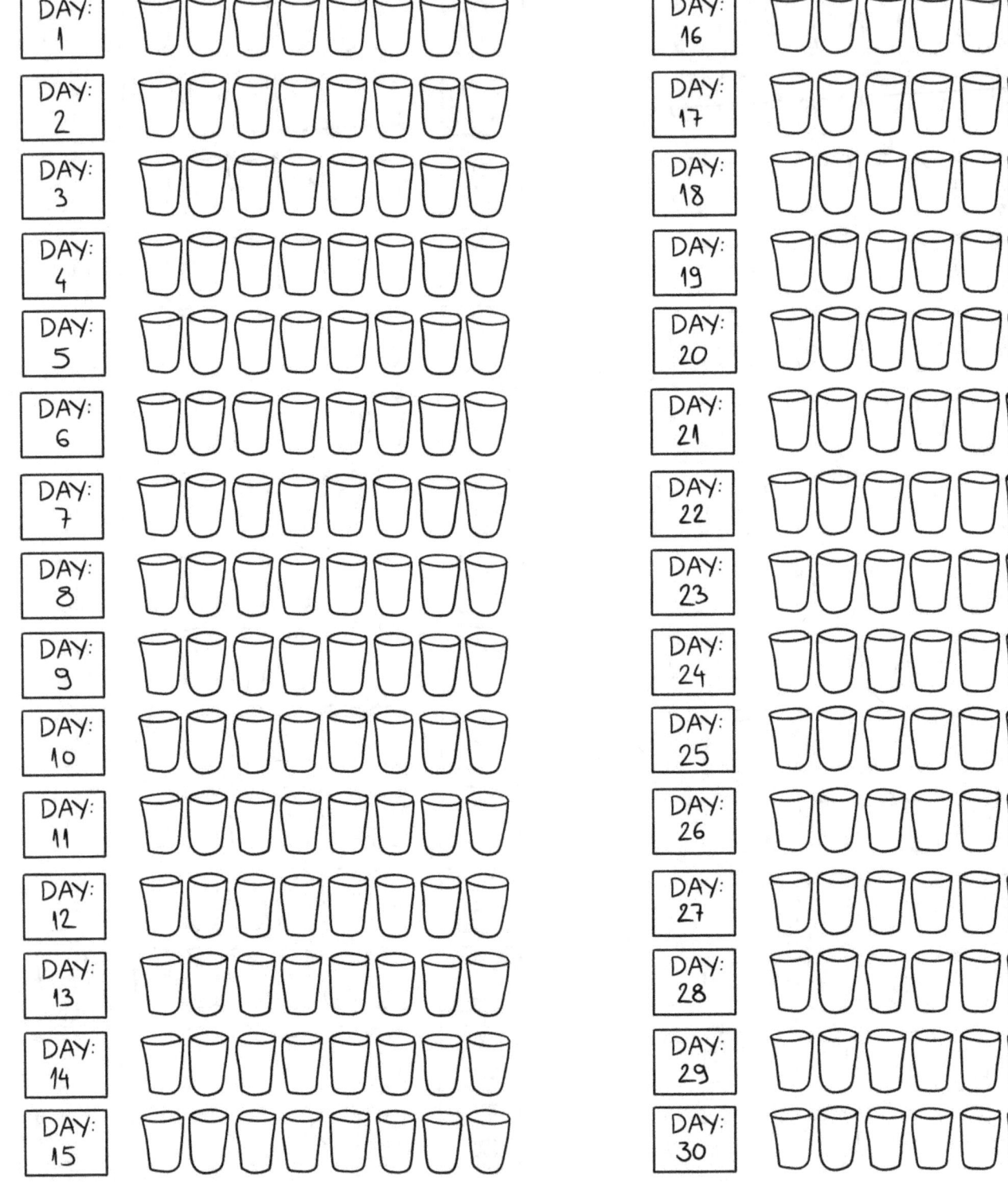

DAY: 1

DAY: 2

DAY: 3

DAY: 4

DAY: 5

DAY: 6

DAY: 7

DAY: 8

DAY: 9

DAY: 10

DAY: 11

DAY: 12

DAY: 13

DAY: 14

DAY: 15

DAY: 16

DAY: 17

DAY: 18

DAY: 19

DAY: 20

DAY: 21

DAY: 22

DAY: 23

DAY: 24

DAY: 25

DAY: 26

DAY: 27

DAY: 28

DAY: 29

DAY: 30

30 DAY WATER challenge

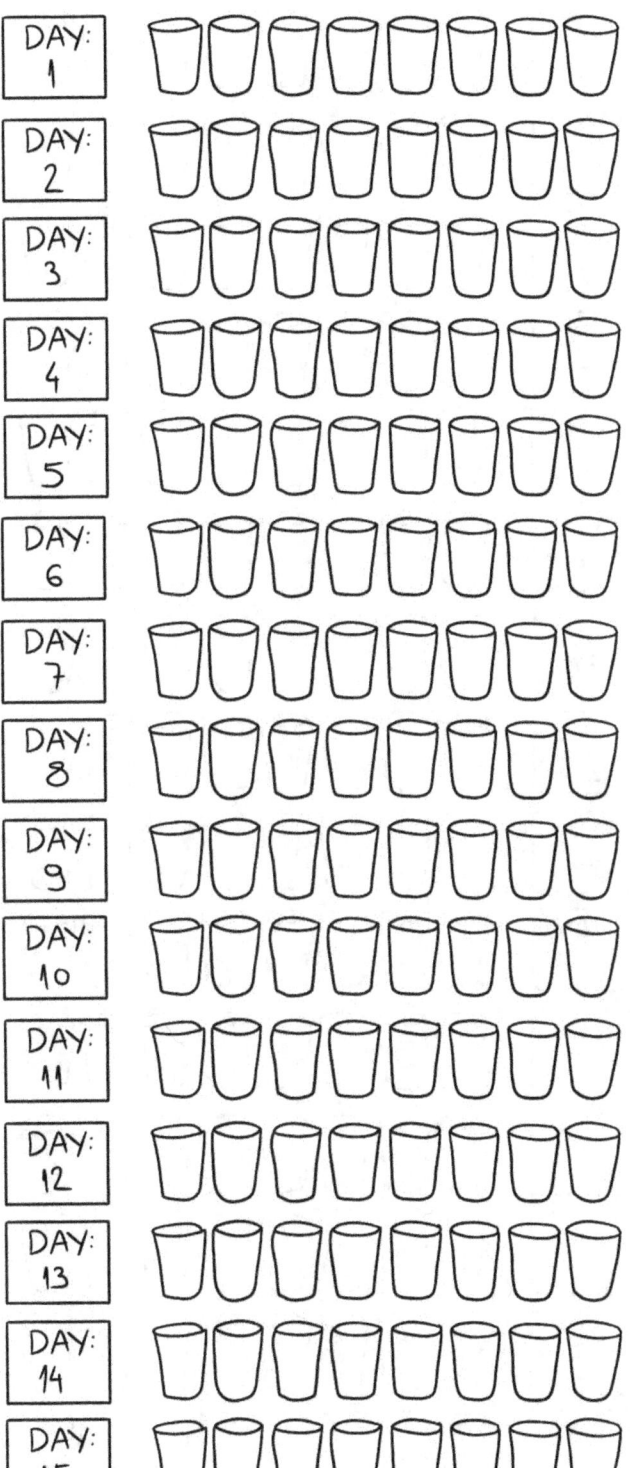

DAY: 1
DAY: 2
DAY: 3
DAY: 4
DAY: 5
DAY: 6
DAY: 7
DAY: 8
DAY: 9
DAY: 10
DAY: 11
DAY: 12
DAY: 13
DAY: 14
DAY: 15

DAY: 16
DAY: 17
DAY: 18
DAY: 19
DAY: 20
DAY: 21
DAY: 22
DAY: 23
DAY: 24
DAY: 25
DAY: 26
DAY: 27
DAY: 28
DAY: 29
DAY: 30

30 DAY
WATER
challenge

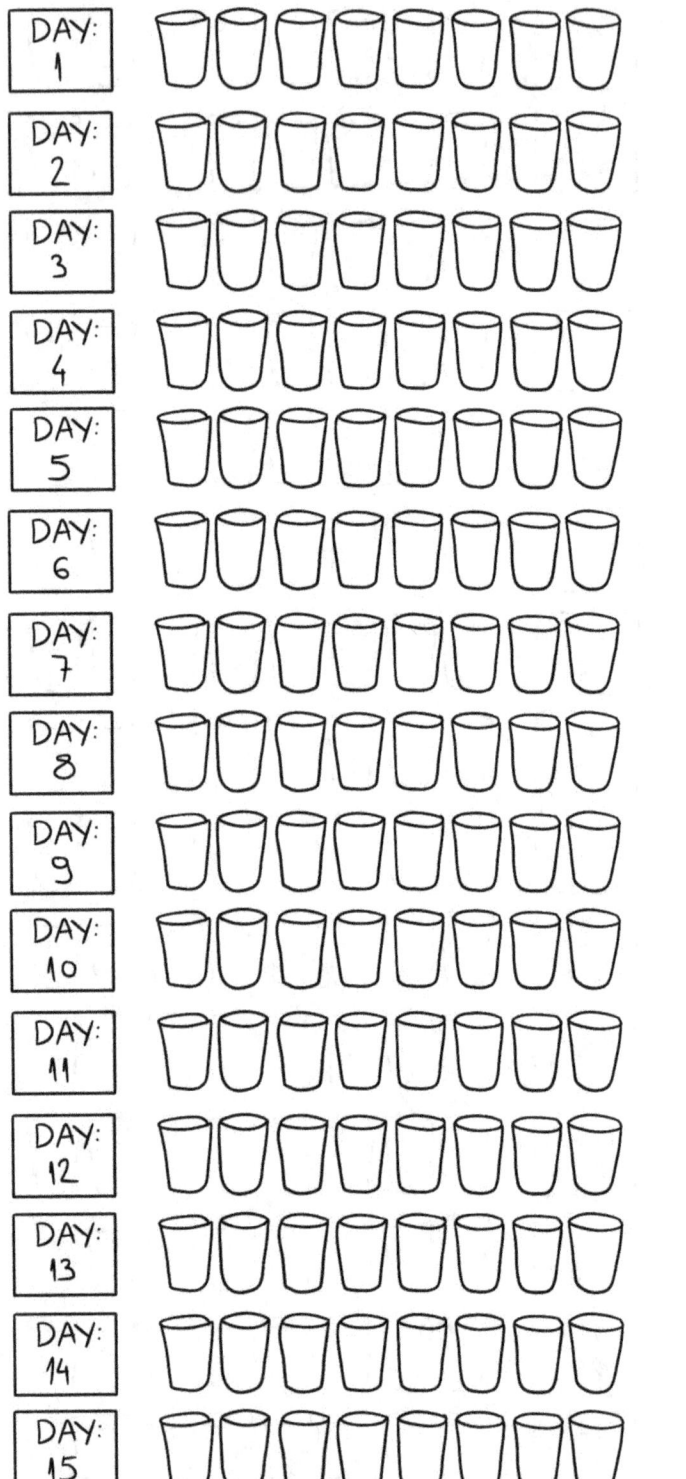

DAY: 1	DAY: 16
DAY: 2	DAY: 17
DAY: 3	DAY: 18
DAY: 4	DAY: 19
DAY: 5	DAY: 20
DAY: 6	DAY: 21
DAY: 7	DAY: 22
DAY: 8	DAY: 23
DAY: 9	DAY: 24
DAY: 10	DAY: 25
DAY: 11	DAY: 26
DAY: 12	DAY: 27
DAY: 13	DAY: 28
DAY: 14	DAY: 29
DAY: 15	DAY: 30

30 DAY
WATER
challenge

DAY: 1	🥛🥛🥛🥛🥛🥛🥛🥛	DAY: 16	🥛🥛🥛🥛🥛🥛🥛🥛
DAY: 2	🥛🥛🥛🥛🥛🥛🥛🥛	DAY: 17	🥛🥛🥛🥛🥛🥛🥛🥛
DAY: 3	🥛🥛🥛🥛🥛🥛🥛🥛	DAY: 18	🥛🥛🥛🥛🥛🥛🥛🥛
DAY: 4	🥛🥛🥛🥛🥛🥛🥛🥛	DAY: 19	🥛🥛🥛🥛🥛🥛🥛🥛
DAY: 5	🥛🥛🥛🥛🥛🥛🥛🥛	DAY: 20	🥛🥛🥛🥛🥛🥛🥛🥛
DAY: 6	🥛🥛🥛🥛🥛🥛🥛🥛	DAY: 21	🥛🥛🥛🥛🥛🥛🥛🥛
DAY: 7	🥛🥛🥛🥛🥛🥛🥛🥛	DAY: 22	🥛🥛🥛🥛🥛🥛🥛🥛
DAY: 8	🥛🥛🥛🥛🥛🥛🥛🥛	DAY: 23	🥛🥛🥛🥛🥛🥛🥛🥛
DAY: 9	🥛🥛🥛🥛🥛🥛🥛🥛	DAY: 24	🥛🥛🥛🥛🥛🥛🥛🥛
DAY: 10	🥛🥛🥛🥛🥛🥛🥛🥛	DAY: 25	🥛🥛🥛🥛🥛🥛🥛🥛
DAY: 11	🥛🥛🥛🥛🥛🥛🥛🥛	DAY: 26	🥛🥛🥛🥛🥛🥛🥛🥛
DAY: 12	🥛🥛🥛🥛🥛🥛🥛🥛	DAY: 27	🥛🥛🥛🥛🥛🥛🥛🥛
DAY: 13	🥛🥛🥛🥛🥛🥛🥛🥛	DAY: 28	🥛🥛🥛🥛🥛🥛🥛🥛
DAY: 14	🥛🥛🥛🥛🥛🥛🥛🥛	DAY: 29	🥛🥛🥛🥛🥛🥛🥛🥛
DAY: 15	🥛🥛🥛🥛🥛🥛🥛🥛	DAY: 30	🥛🥛🥛🥛🥛🥛🥛🥛

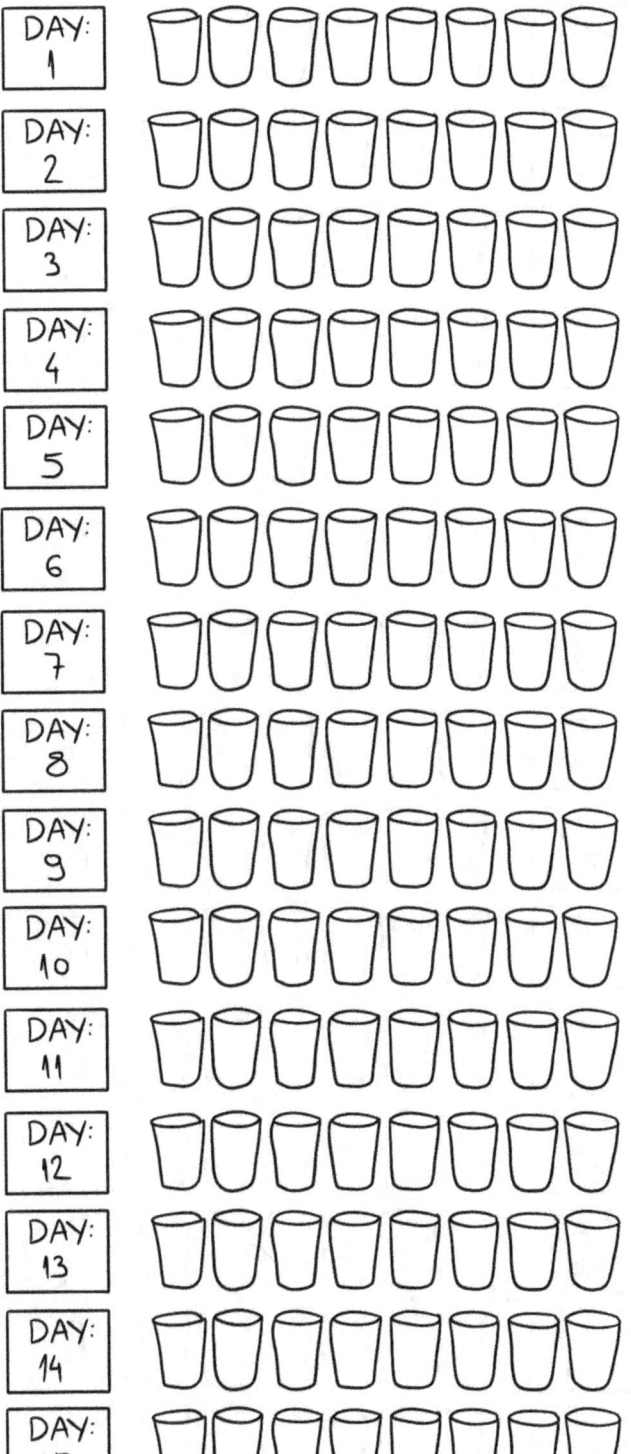

30 DAY
WATER
challenge

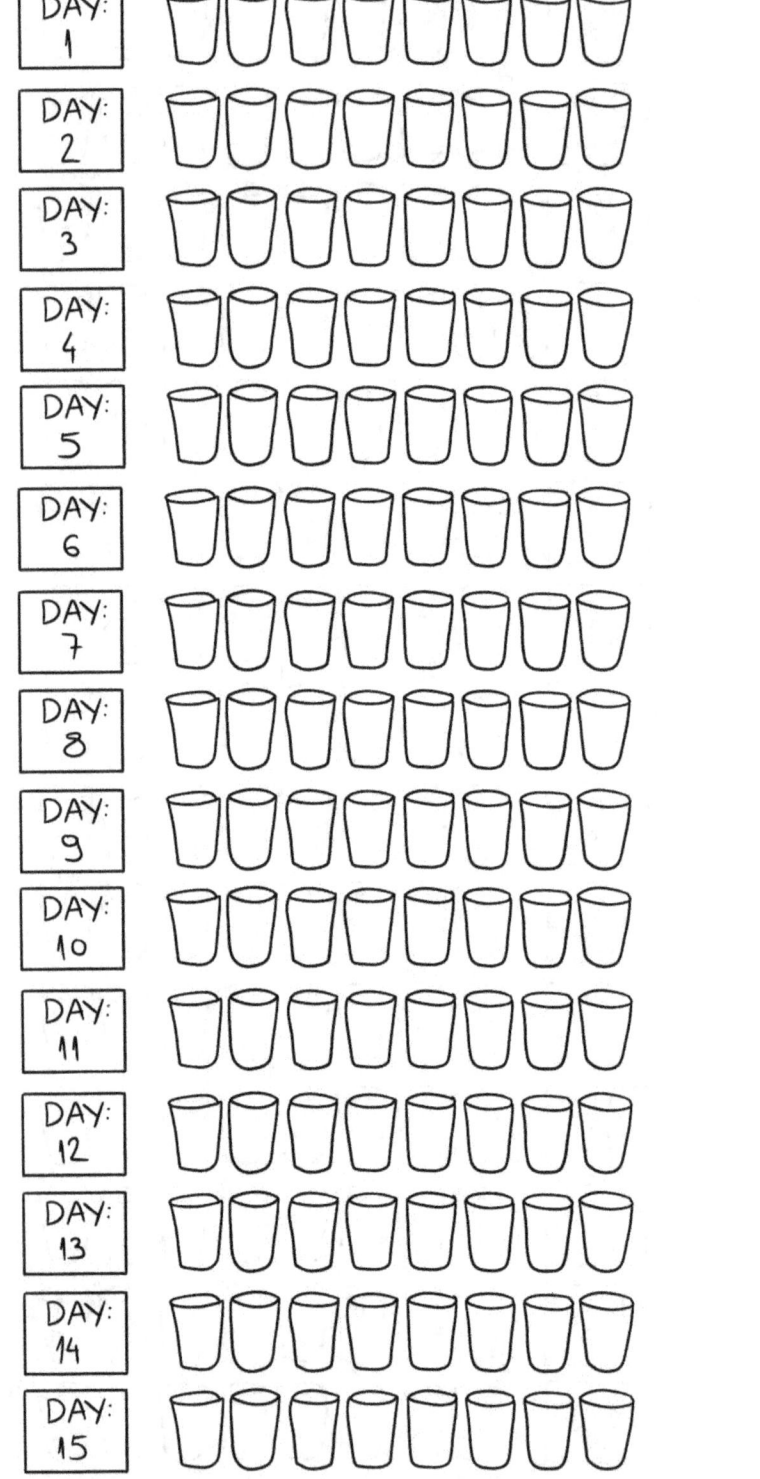

DAY: 1								
DAY: 2								
DAY: 3								
DAY: 4								
DAY: 5								
DAY: 6								
DAY: 7								
DAY: 8								
DAY: 9								
DAY: 10								
DAY: 11								
DAY: 12								
DAY: 13								
DAY: 14								
DAY: 15								

DAY: 16								
DAY: 17								
DAY: 18								
DAY: 19								
DAY: 20								
DAY: 21								
DAY: 22								
DAY: 23								
DAY: 24								
DAY: 25								
DAY: 26								
DAY: 27								
DAY: 28								
DAY: 29								
DAY: 30								

30 DAY WATER challenge

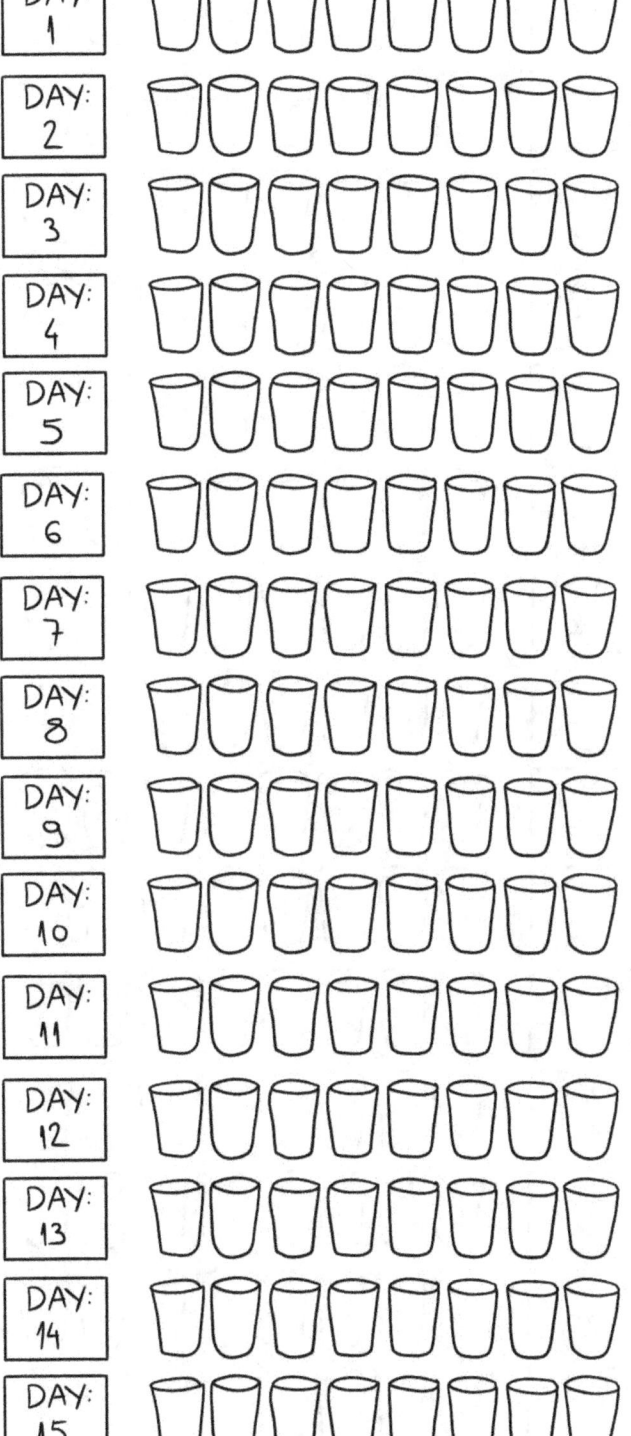

DAY: 1	🥛🥛🥛🥛🥛🥛🥛🥛
DAY: 2	🥛🥛🥛🥛🥛🥛🥛🥛
DAY: 3	🥛🥛🥛🥛🥛🥛🥛🥛
DAY: 4	🥛🥛🥛🥛🥛🥛🥛🥛
DAY: 5	🥛🥛🥛🥛🥛🥛🥛🥛
DAY: 6	🥛🥛🥛🥛🥛🥛🥛🥛
DAY: 7	🥛🥛🥛🥛🥛🥛🥛🥛
DAY: 8	🥛🥛🥛🥛🥛🥛🥛🥛
DAY: 9	🥛🥛🥛🥛🥛🥛🥛🥛
DAY: 10	🥛🥛🥛🥛🥛🥛🥛🥛
DAY: 11	🥛🥛🥛🥛🥛🥛🥛🥛
DAY: 12	🥛🥛🥛🥛🥛🥛🥛🥛
DAY: 13	🥛🥛🥛🥛🥛🥛🥛🥛
DAY: 14	🥛🥛🥛🥛🥛🥛🥛🥛
DAY: 15	🥛🥛🥛🥛🥛🥛🥛🥛

DAY: 16	🥛🥛🥛🥛🥛🥛🥛🥛
DAY: 17	🥛🥛🥛🥛🥛🥛🥛🥛
DAY: 18	🥛🥛🥛🥛🥛🥛🥛🥛
DAY: 19	🥛🥛🥛🥛🥛🥛🥛🥛
DAY: 20	🥛🥛🥛🥛🥛🥛🥛🥛
DAY: 21	🥛🥛🥛🥛🥛🥛🥛🥛
DAY: 22	🥛🥛🥛🥛🥛🥛🥛🥛
DAY: 23	🥛🥛🥛🥛🥛🥛🥛🥛
DAY: 24	🥛🥛🥛🥛🥛🥛🥛🥛
DAY: 25	🥛🥛🥛🥛🥛🥛🥛🥛
DAY: 26	🥛🥛🥛🥛🥛🥛🥛🥛
DAY: 27	🥛🥛🥛🥛🥛🥛🥛🥛
DAY: 28	🥛🥛🥛🥛🥛🥛🥛🥛
DAY: 29	🥛🥛🥛🥛🥛🥛🥛🥛
DAY: 30	🥛🥛🥛🥛🥛🥛🥛🥛

30 DAY WATER challenge

DAY: 1	DAY: 16
DAY: 2	DAY: 17
DAY: 3	DAY: 18
DAY: 4	DAY: 19
DAY: 5	DAY: 20
DAY: 6	DAY: 21
DAY: 7	DAY: 22
DAY: 8	DAY: 23
DAY: 9	DAY: 24
DAY: 10	DAY: 25
DAY: 11	DAY: 26
DAY: 12	DAY: 27
DAY: 13	DAY: 28
DAY: 14	DAY: 29
DAY: 15	DAY: 30

30 DAY
WATER
challenge

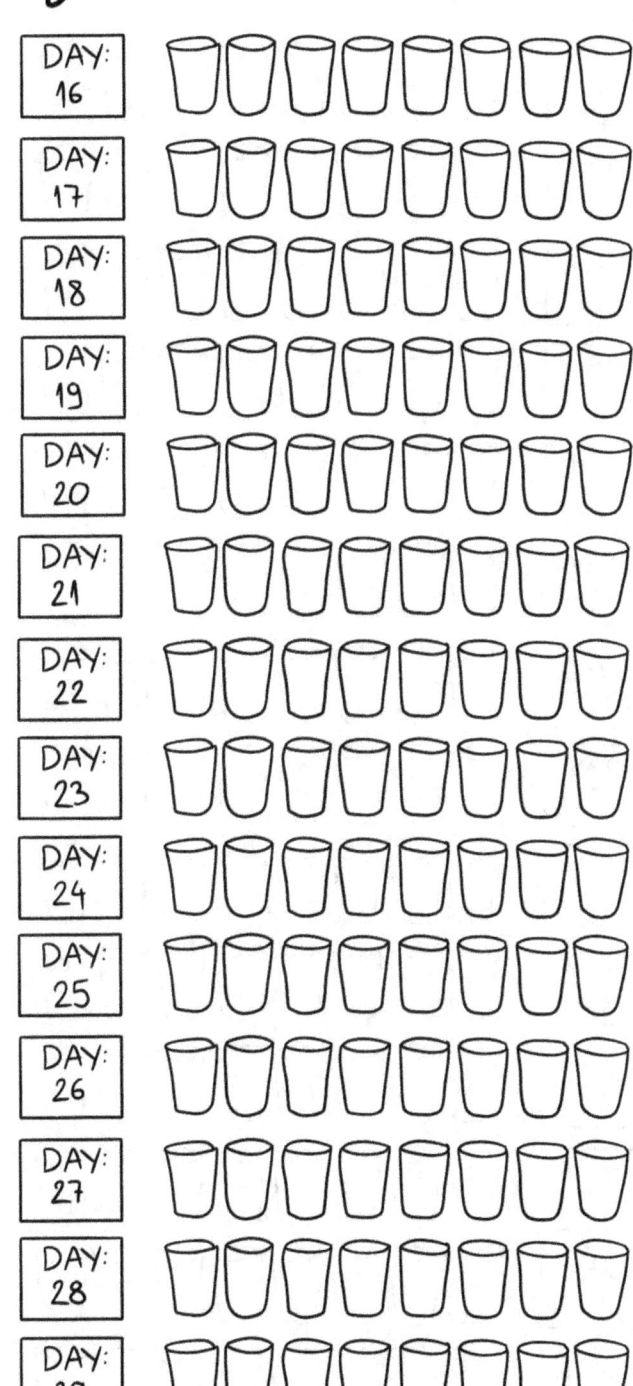

DAY: 1	🥛🥛🥛🥛🥛🥛🥛🥛
DAY: 2	🥛🥛🥛🥛🥛🥛🥛🥛
DAY: 3	🥛🥛🥛🥛🥛🥛🥛🥛
DAY: 4	🥛🥛🥛🥛🥛🥛🥛🥛
DAY: 5	🥛🥛🥛🥛🥛🥛🥛🥛
DAY: 6	🥛🥛🥛🥛🥛🥛🥛🥛
DAY: 7	🥛🥛🥛🥛🥛🥛🥛🥛
DAY: 8	🥛🥛🥛🥛🥛🥛🥛🥛
DAY: 9	🥛🥛🥛🥛🥛🥛🥛🥛
DAY: 10	🥛🥛🥛🥛🥛🥛🥛🥛
DAY: 11	🥛🥛🥛🥛🥛🥛🥛🥛
DAY: 12	🥛🥛🥛🥛🥛🥛🥛🥛
DAY: 13	🥛🥛🥛🥛🥛🥛🥛🥛
DAY: 14	🥛🥛🥛🥛🥛🥛🥛🥛
DAY: 15	🥛🥛🥛🥛🥛🥛🥛🥛
DAY: 16	🥛🥛🥛🥛🥛🥛🥛🥛
DAY: 17	🥛🥛🥛🥛🥛🥛🥛🥛
DAY: 18	🥛🥛🥛🥛🥛🥛🥛🥛
DAY: 19	🥛🥛🥛🥛🥛🥛🥛🥛
DAY: 20	🥛🥛🥛🥛🥛🥛🥛🥛
DAY: 21	🥛🥛🥛🥛🥛🥛🥛🥛
DAY: 22	🥛🥛🥛🥛🥛🥛🥛🥛
DAY: 23	🥛🥛🥛🥛🥛🥛🥛🥛
DAY: 24	🥛🥛🥛🥛🥛🥛🥛🥛
DAY: 25	🥛🥛🥛🥛🥛🥛🥛🥛
DAY: 26	🥛🥛🥛🥛🥛🥛🥛🥛
DAY: 27	🥛🥛🥛🥛🥛🥛🥛🥛
DAY: 28	🥛🥛🥛🥛🥛🥛🥛🥛
DAY: 29	🥛🥛🥛🥛🥛🥛🥛🥛
DAY: 30	🥛🥛🥛🥛🥛🥛🥛🥛

30 DAY
WATER
challenge

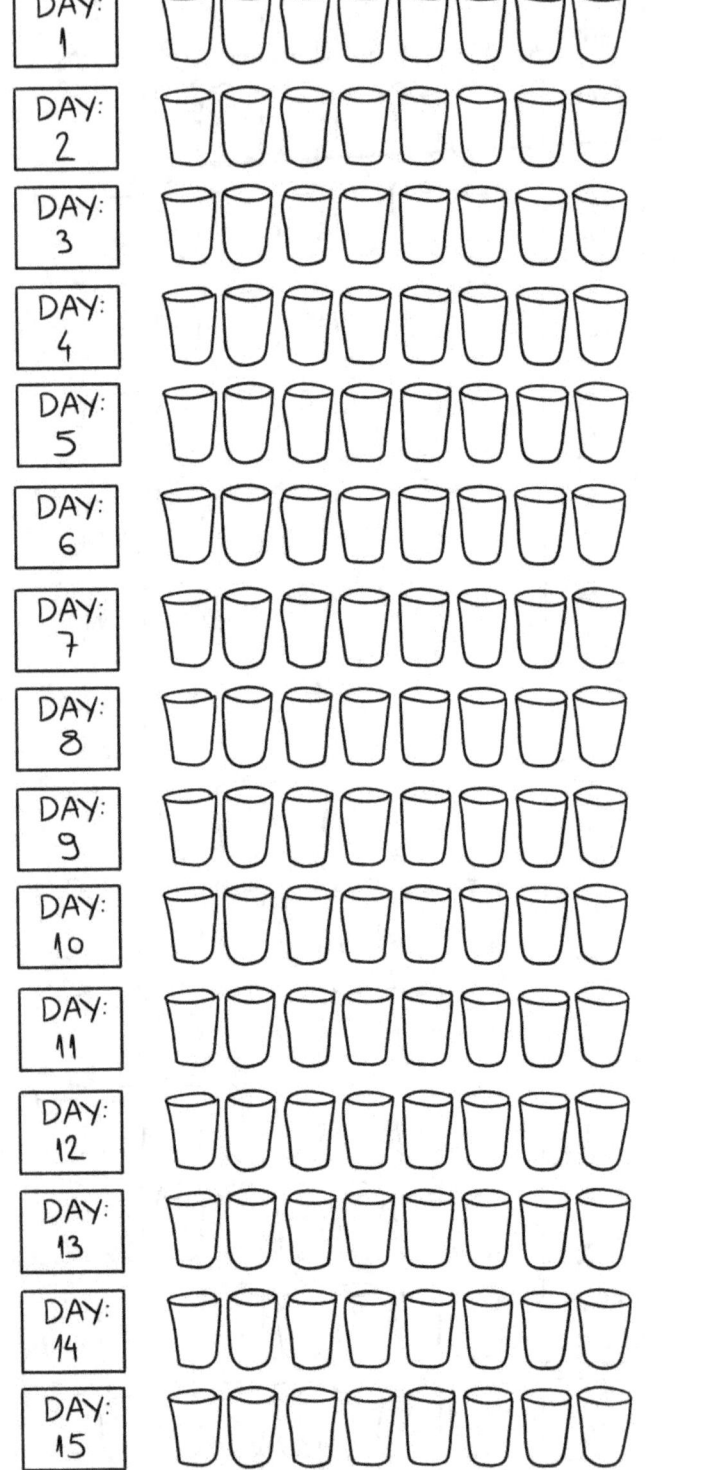

DAY: 1							
DAY: 2							
DAY: 3							
DAY: 4							
DAY: 5							
DAY: 6							
DAY: 7							
DAY: 8							
DAY: 9							
DAY: 10							
DAY: 11							
DAY: 12							
DAY: 13							
DAY: 14							
DAY: 15							

DAY: 16							
DAY: 17							
DAY: 18							
DAY: 19							
DAY: 20							
DAY: 21							
DAY: 22							
DAY: 23							
DAY: 24							
DAY: 25							
DAY: 26							
DAY: 27							
DAY: 28							
DAY: 29							
DAY: 30							

30 DAY
WATER
challenge

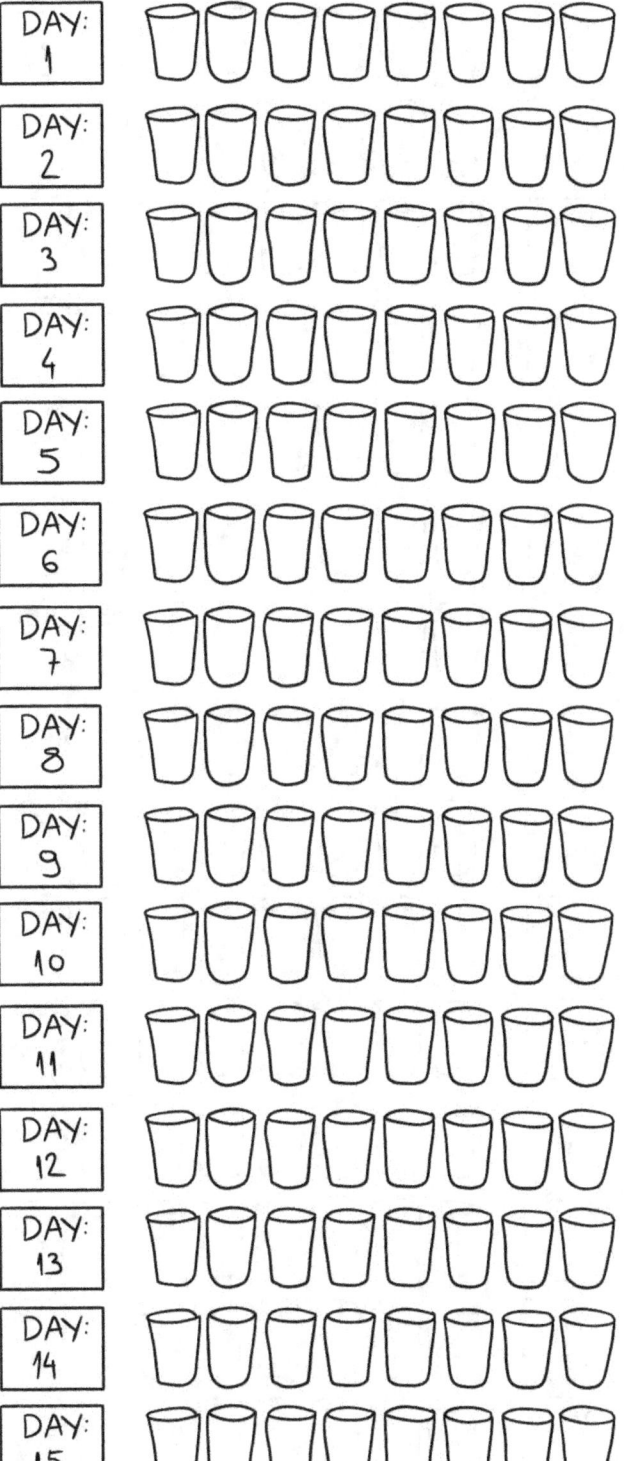

DAY: 1								DAY: 16							
DAY: 2								DAY: 17							
DAY: 3								DAY: 18							
DAY: 4								DAY: 19							
DAY: 5								DAY: 20							
DAY: 6								DAY: 21							
DAY: 7								DAY: 22							
DAY: 8								DAY: 23							
DAY: 9								DAY: 24							
DAY: 10								DAY: 25							
DAY: 11								DAY: 26							
DAY: 12								DAY: 27							
DAY: 13								DAY: 28							
DAY: 14								DAY: 29							
DAY: 15								DAY: 30							

30 DAY
WATER
challenge

DAY: 1	□□□□□□□□
DAY: 2	□□□□□□□□
DAY: 3	□□□□□□□□
DAY: 4	□□□□□□□□
DAY: 5	□□□□□□□□
DAY: 6	□□□□□□□□
DAY: 7	□□□□□□□□
DAY: 8	□□□□□□□□
DAY: 9	□□□□□□□□
DAY: 10	□□□□□□□□
DAY: 11	□□□□□□□□
DAY: 12	□□□□□□□□
DAY: 13	□□□□□□□□
DAY: 14	□□□□□□□□
DAY: 15	□□□□□□□□

DAY: 16	□□□□□□□□
DAY: 17	□□□□□□□□
DAY: 18	□□□□□□□□
DAY: 19	□□□□□□□□
DAY: 20	□□□□□□□□
DAY: 21	□□□□□□□□
DAY: 22	□□□□□□□□
DAY: 23	□□□□□□□□
DAY: 24	□□□□□□□□
DAY: 25	□□□□□□□□
DAY: 26	□□□□□□□□
DAY: 27	□□□□□□□□
DAY: 28	□□□□□□□□
DAY: 29	□□□□□□□□
DAY: 30	□□□□□□□□

30 DAY
WATER
challenge

DAY: 1	DAY: 16
DAY: 2	DAY: 17
DAY: 3	DAY: 18
DAY: 4	DAY: 19
DAY: 5	DAY: 20
DAY: 6	DAY: 21
DAY: 7	DAY: 22
DAY: 8	DAY: 23
DAY: 9	DAY: 24
DAY: 10	DAY: 25
DAY: 11	DAY: 26
DAY: 12	DAY: 27
DAY: 13	DAY: 28
DAY: 14	DAY: 29
DAY: 15	DAY: 30

30 DAY WATER challenge

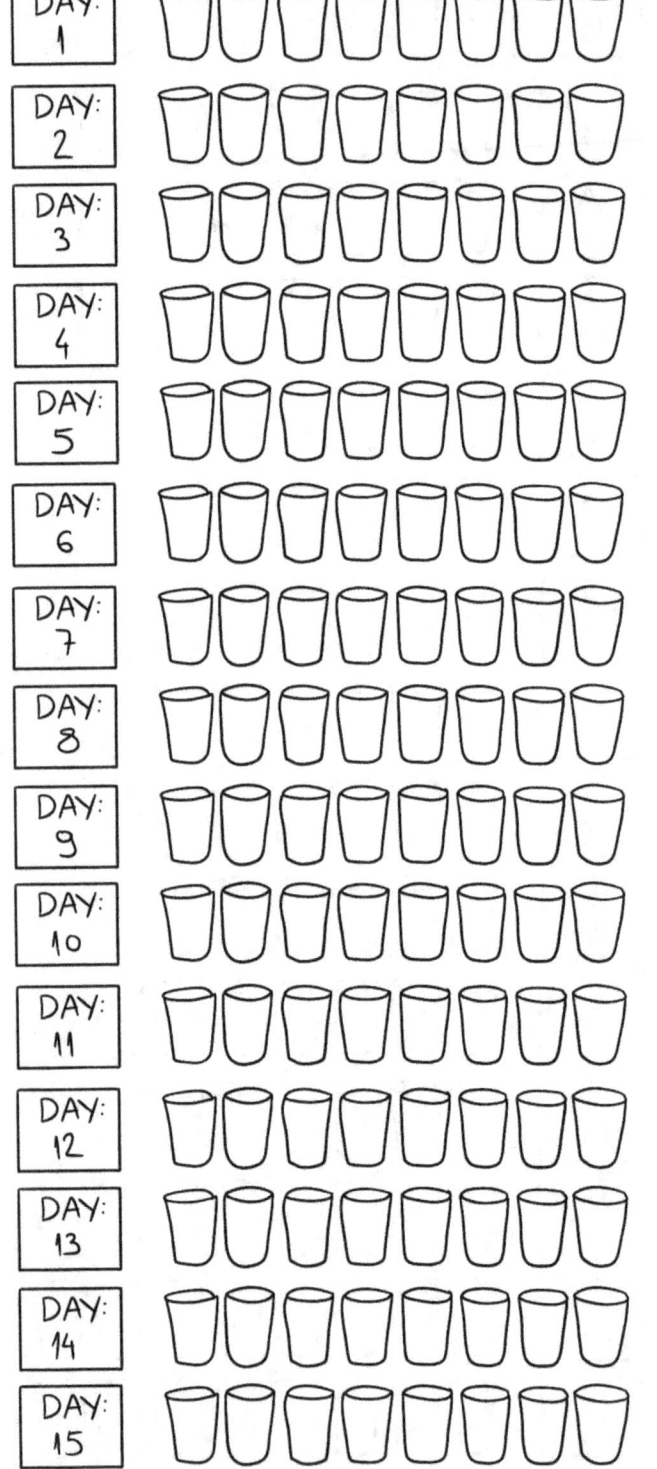

DAY: 1								
DAY: 2								
DAY: 3								
DAY: 4								
DAY: 5								
DAY: 6								
DAY: 7								
DAY: 8								
DAY: 9								
DAY: 10								
DAY: 11								
DAY: 12								
DAY: 13								
DAY: 14								
DAY: 15								

DAY: 16								
DAY: 17								
DAY: 18								
DAY: 19								
DAY: 20								
DAY: 21								
DAY: 22								
DAY: 23								
DAY: 24								
DAY: 25								
DAY: 26								
DAY: 27								
DAY: 28								
DAY: 29								
DAY: 30								

30 DAY
WATER
challenge

DAY: 1								
DAY: 2								
DAY: 3								
DAY: 4								
DAY: 5								
DAY: 6								
DAY: 7								
DAY: 8								
DAY: 9								
DAY: 10								
DAY: 11								
DAY: 12								
DAY: 13								
DAY: 14								
DAY: 15								

DAY: 16								
DAY: 17								
DAY: 18								
DAY: 19								
DAY: 20								
DAY: 21								
DAY: 22								
DAY: 23								
DAY: 24								
DAY: 25								
DAY: 26								
DAY: 27								
DAY: 28								
DAY: 29								
DAY: 30								

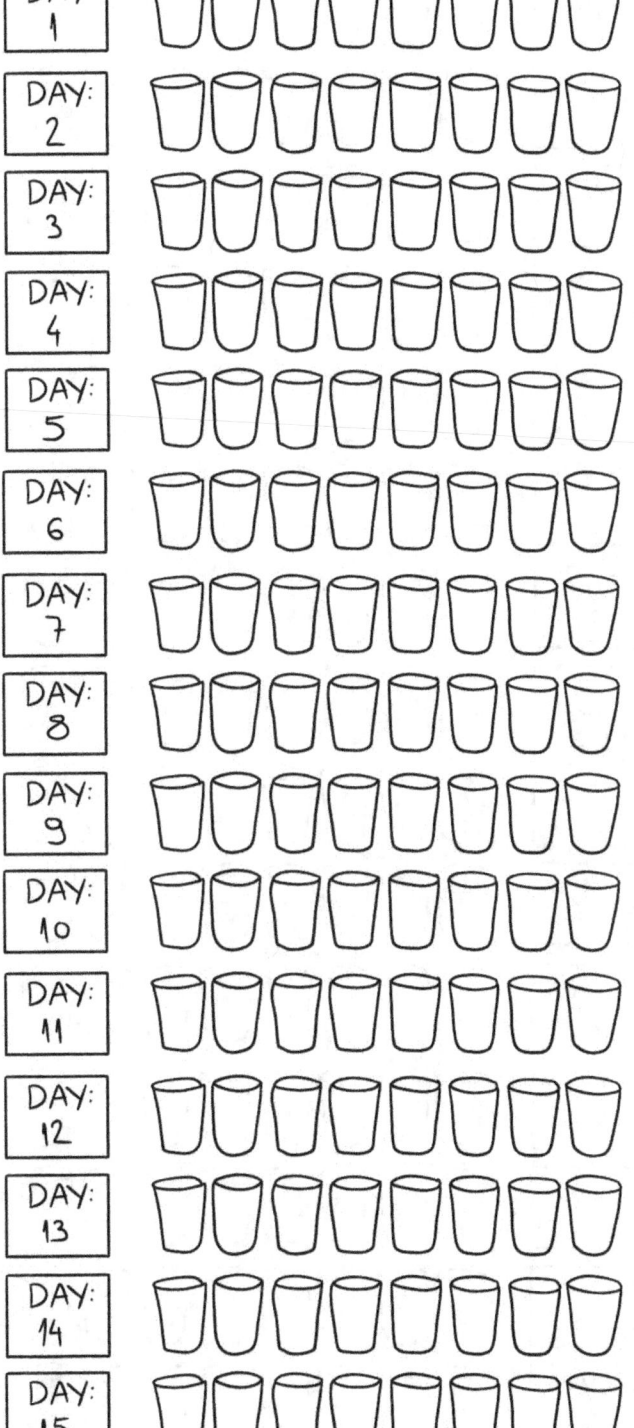

30 DAY
WATER
challenge

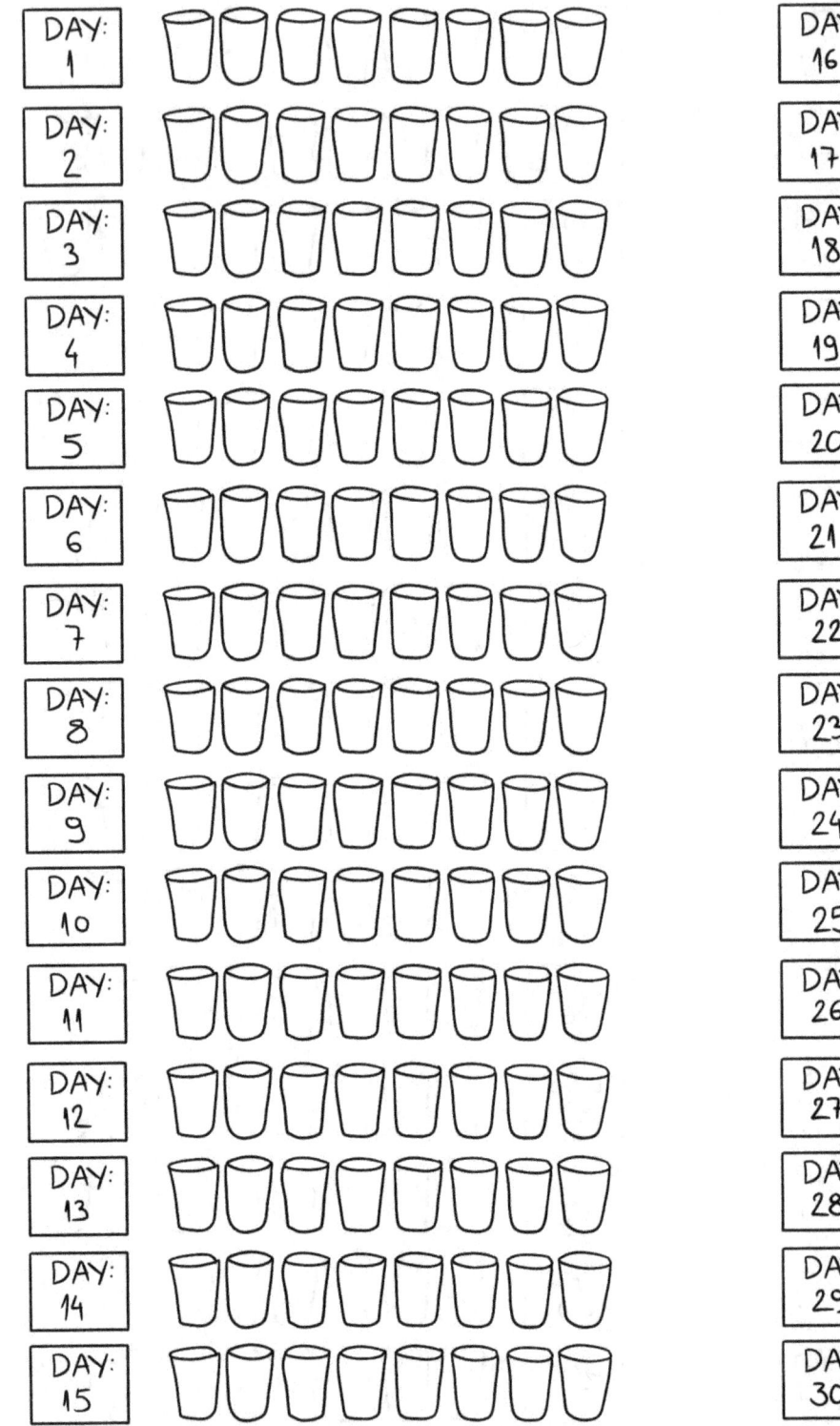

DAY: 1								
DAY: 2								
DAY: 3								
DAY: 4								
DAY: 5								
DAY: 6								
DAY: 7								
DAY: 8								
DAY: 9								
DAY: 10								
DAY: 11								
DAY: 12								
DAY: 13								
DAY: 14								
DAY: 15								

DAY: 16								
DAY: 17								
DAY: 18								
DAY: 19								
DAY: 20								
DAY: 21								
DAY: 22								
DAY: 23								
DAY: 24								
DAY: 25								
DAY: 26								
DAY: 27								
DAY: 28								
DAY: 29								
DAY: 30								

30 DAY WATER *challenge*

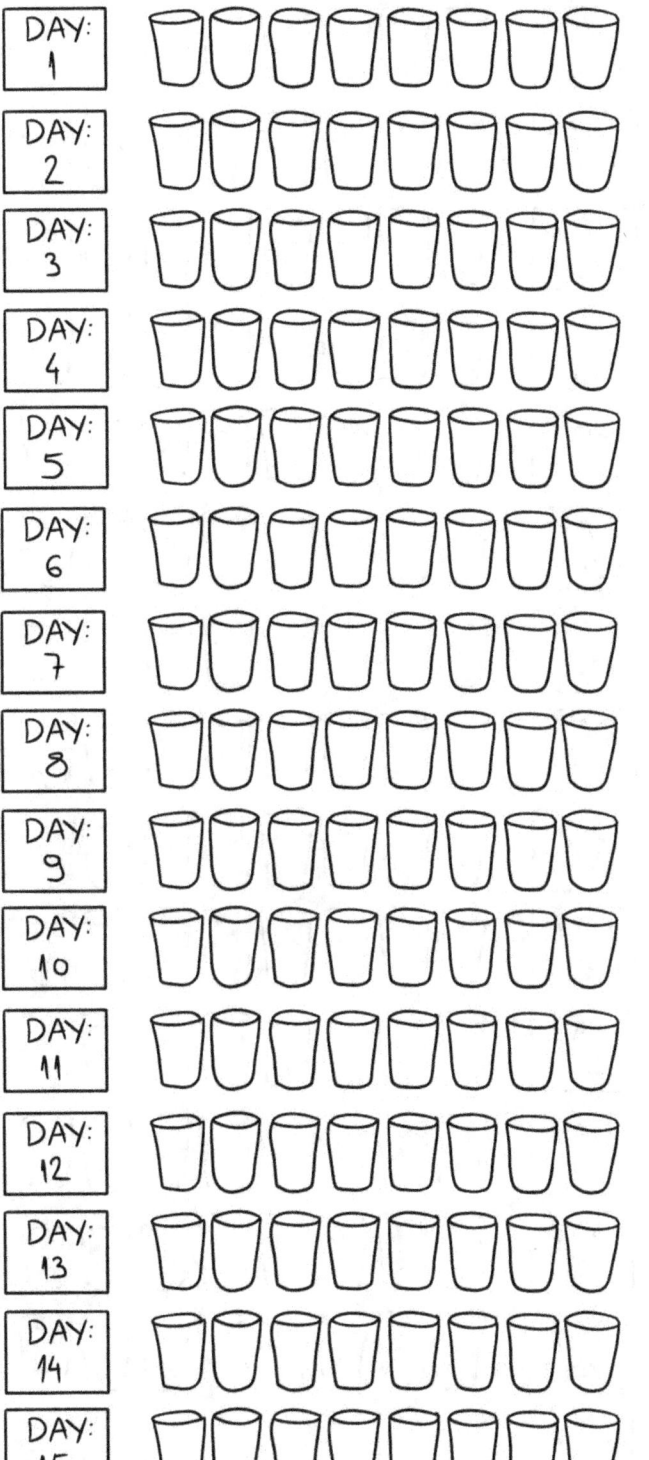

DAY: 1		DAY: 16
DAY: 2		DAY: 17
DAY: 3		DAY: 18
DAY: 4		DAY: 19
DAY: 5		DAY: 20
DAY: 6		DAY: 21
DAY: 7		DAY: 22
DAY: 8		DAY: 23
DAY: 9		DAY: 24
DAY: 10		DAY: 25
DAY: 11		DAY: 26
DAY: 12		DAY: 27
DAY: 13		DAY: 28
DAY: 14		DAY: 29
DAY: 15		DAY: 30

30 DAY
WATER
challenge

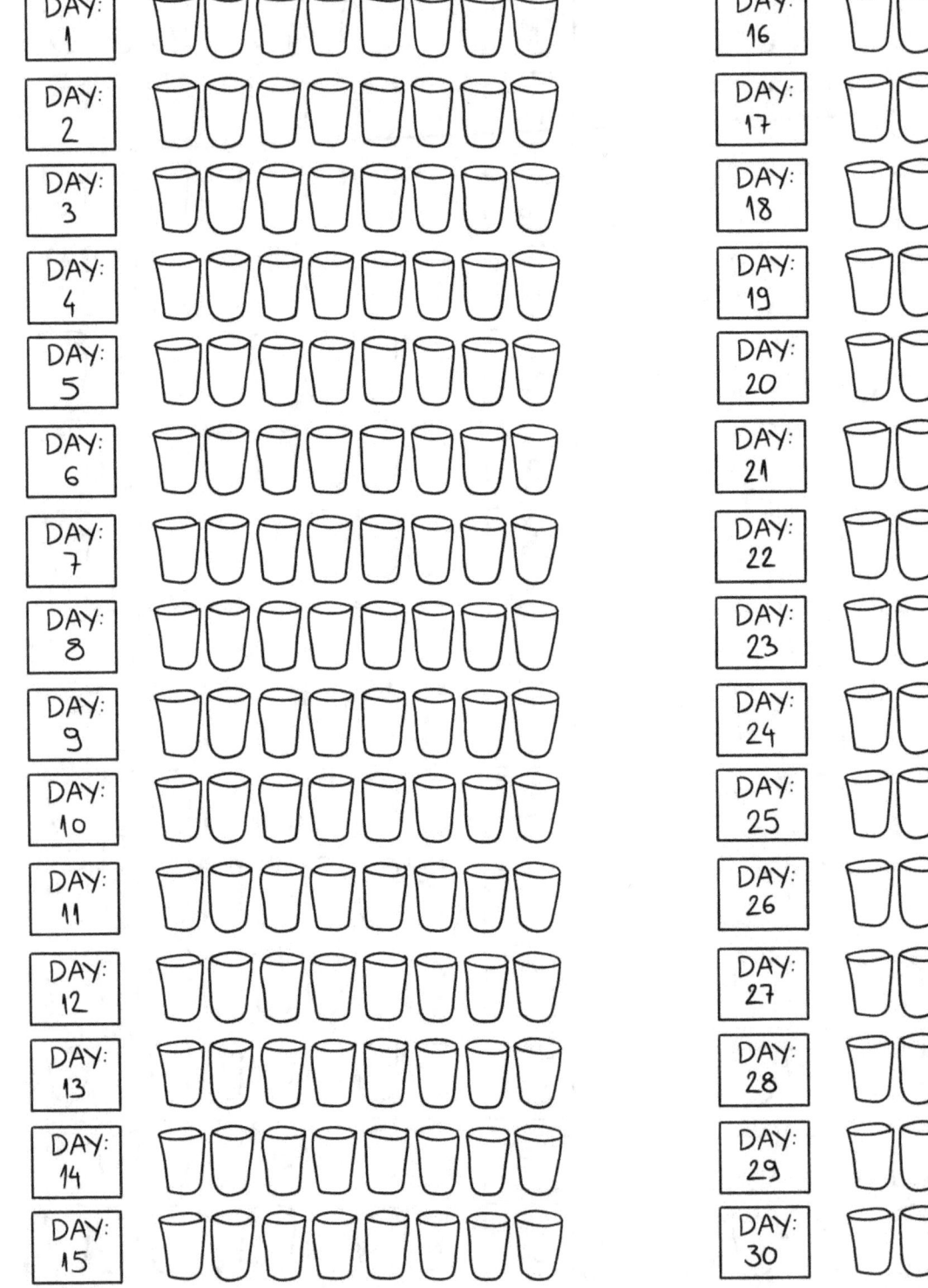

30 DAY
WATER
challenge

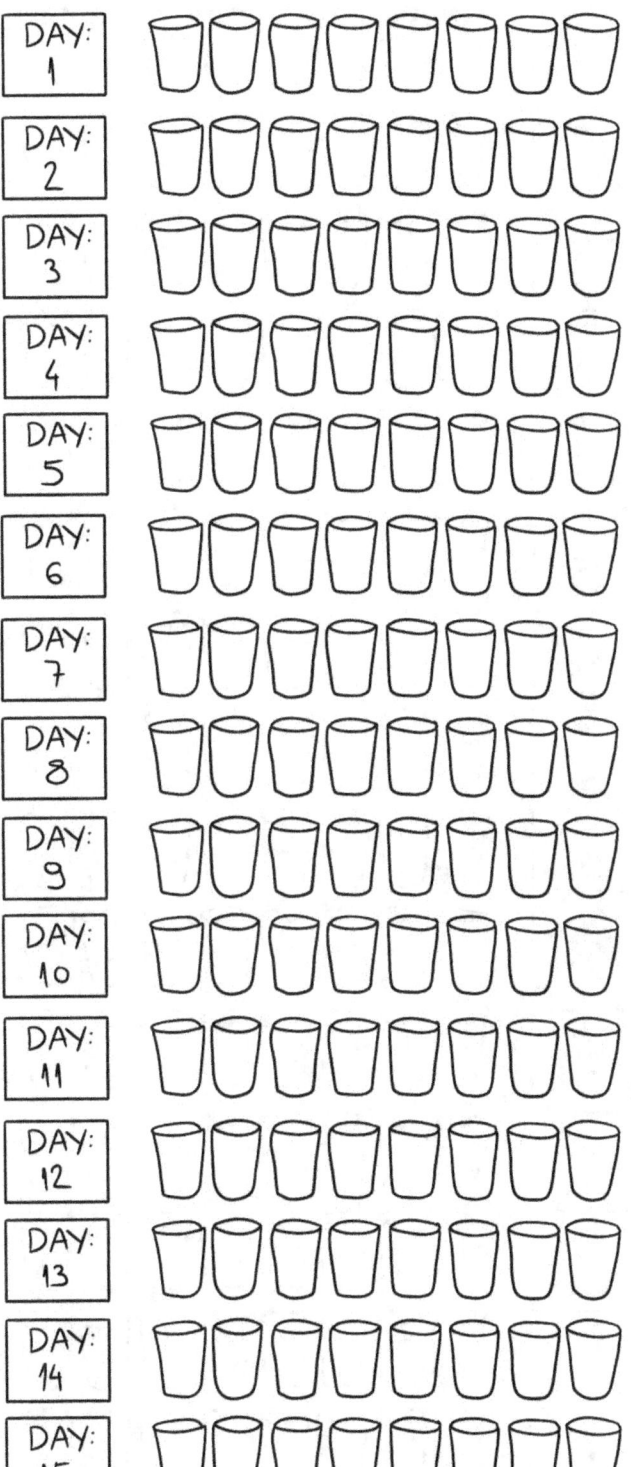

DAY: 1	☐☐☐☐☐☐☐☐
DAY: 2	☐☐☐☐☐☐☐☐
DAY: 3	☐☐☐☐☐☐☐☐
DAY: 4	☐☐☐☐☐☐☐☐
DAY: 5	☐☐☐☐☐☐☐☐
DAY: 6	☐☐☐☐☐☐☐☐
DAY: 7	☐☐☐☐☐☐☐☐
DAY: 8	☐☐☐☐☐☐☐☐
DAY: 9	☐☐☐☐☐☐☐☐
DAY: 10	☐☐☐☐☐☐☐☐
DAY: 11	☐☐☐☐☐☐☐☐
DAY: 12	☐☐☐☐☐☐☐☐
DAY: 13	☐☐☐☐☐☐☐☐
DAY: 14	☐☐☐☐☐☐☐☐
DAY: 15	☐☐☐☐☐☐☐☐

DAY: 16	☐☐☐☐☐☐☐☐
DAY: 17	☐☐☐☐☐☐☐☐
DAY: 18	☐☐☐☐☐☐☐☐
DAY: 19	☐☐☐☐☐☐☐☐
DAY: 20	☐☐☐☐☐☐☐☐
DAY: 21	☐☐☐☐☐☐☐☐
DAY: 22	☐☐☐☐☐☐☐☐
DAY: 23	☐☐☐☐☐☐☐☐
DAY: 24	☐☐☐☐☐☐☐☐
DAY: 25	☐☐☐☐☐☐☐☐
DAY: 26	☐☐☐☐☐☐☐☐
DAY: 27	☐☐☐☐☐☐☐☐
DAY: 28	☐☐☐☐☐☐☐☐
DAY: 29	☐☐☐☐☐☐☐☐
DAY: 30	☐☐☐☐☐☐☐☐

30 DAY
WATER
challenge

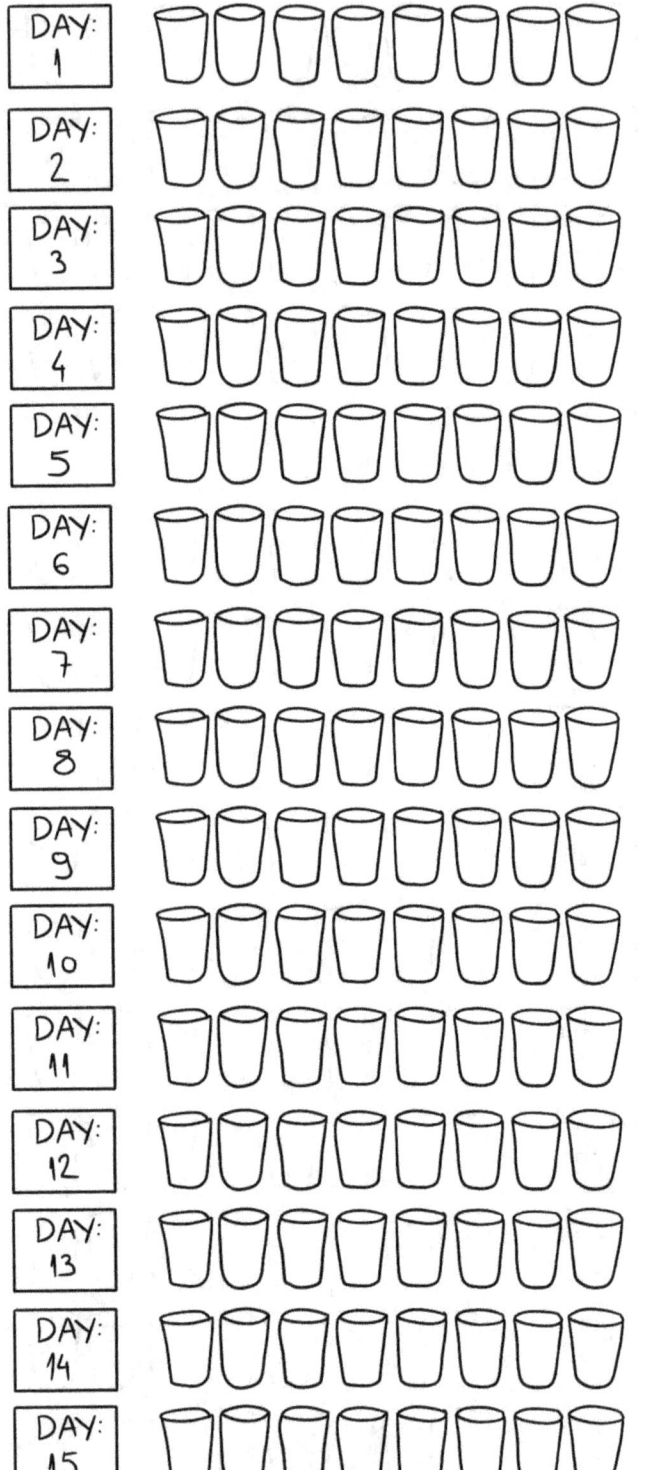

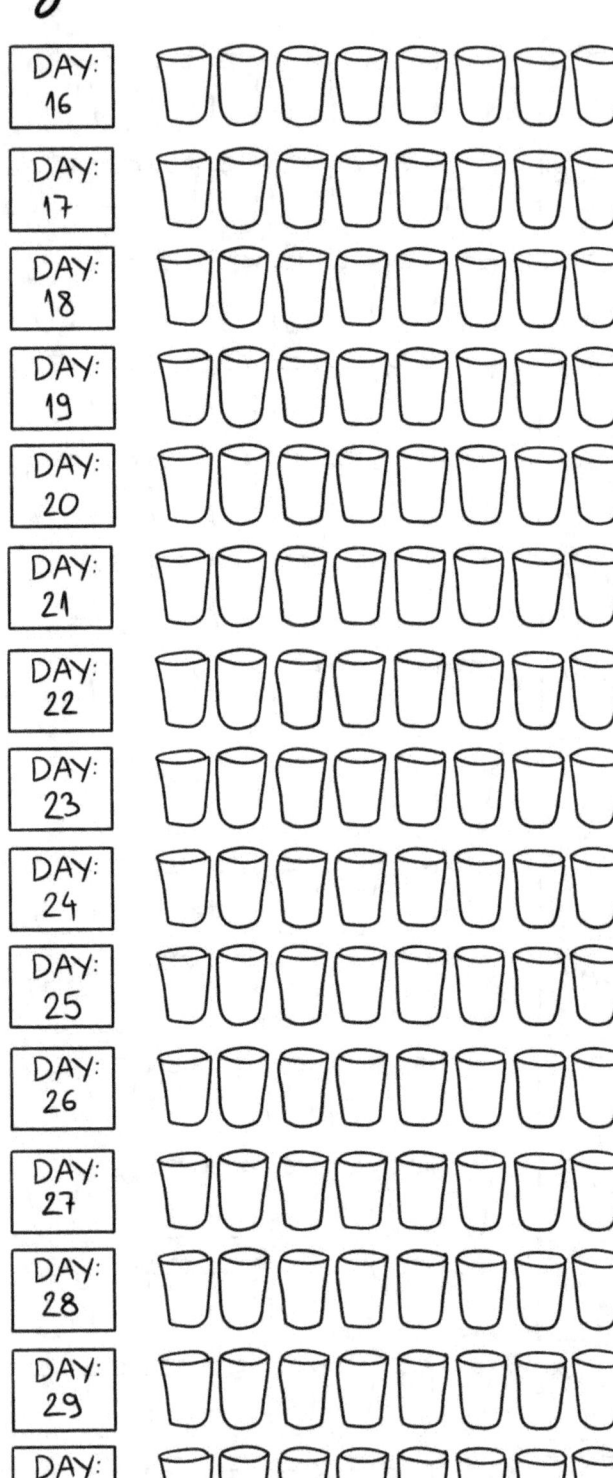

DAY: 1	DAY: 16
DAY: 2	DAY: 17
DAY: 3	DAY: 18
DAY: 4	DAY: 19
DAY: 5	DAY: 20
DAY: 6	DAY: 21
DAY: 7	DAY: 22
DAY: 8	DAY: 23
DAY: 9	DAY: 24
DAY: 10	DAY: 25
DAY: 11	DAY: 26
DAY: 12	DAY: 27
DAY: 13	DAY: 28
DAY: 14	DAY: 29
DAY: 15	DAY: 30

30 DAY
WATER
challenge

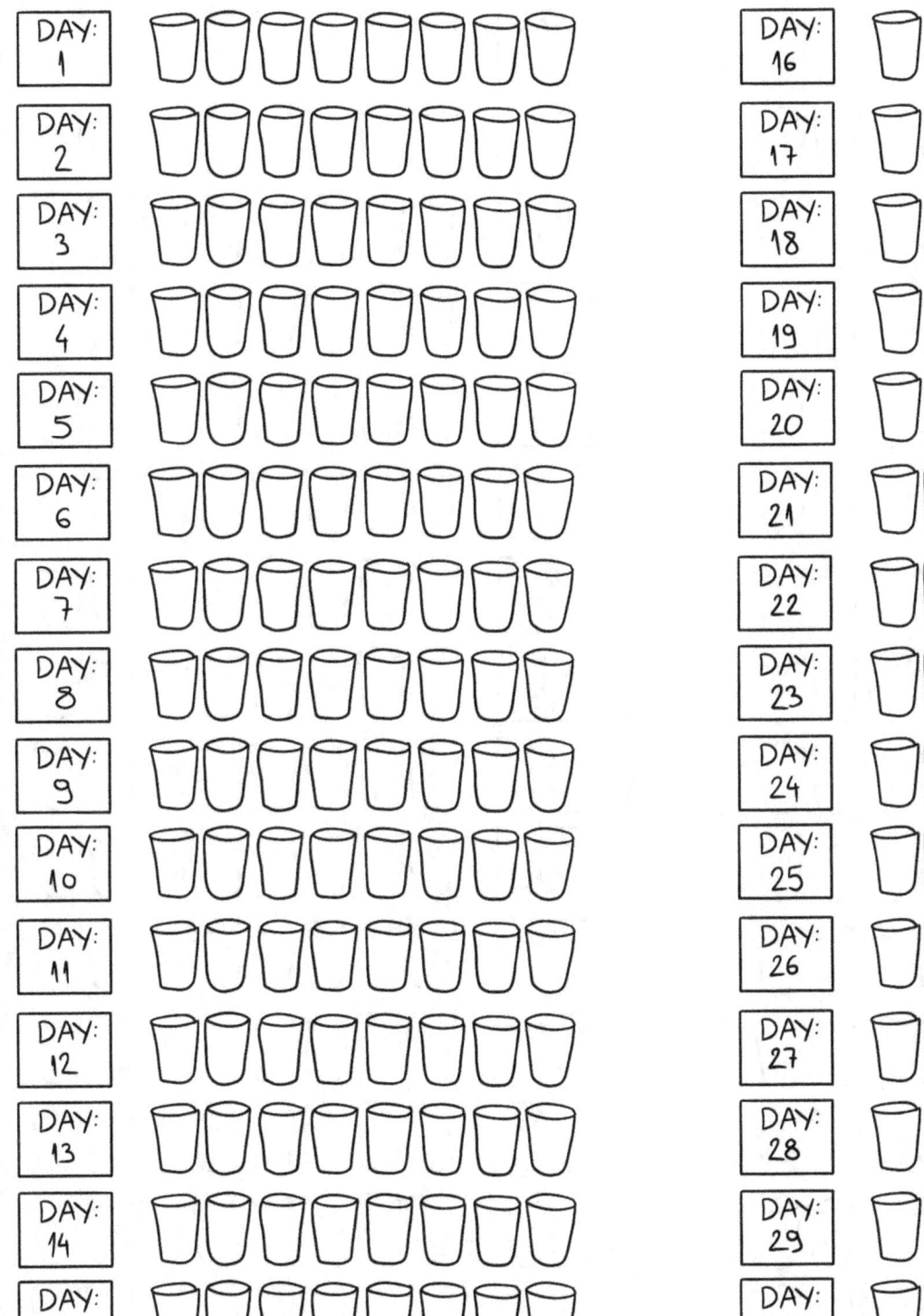

DAY: 1								DAY: 16							
DAY: 2								DAY: 17							
DAY: 3								DAY: 18							
DAY: 4								DAY: 19							
DAY: 5								DAY: 20							
DAY: 6								DAY: 21							
DAY: 7								DAY: 22							
DAY: 8								DAY: 23							
DAY: 9								DAY: 24							
DAY: 10								DAY: 25							
DAY: 11								DAY: 26							
DAY: 12								DAY: 27							
DAY: 13								DAY: 28							
DAY: 14								DAY: 29							
DAY: 15								DAY: 30							

30 DAY WATER challenge

DAY: 1									DAY: 16							
DAY: 2									DAY: 17							
DAY: 3									DAY: 18							
DAY: 4									DAY: 19							
DAY: 5									DAY: 20							
DAY: 6									DAY: 21							
DAY: 7									DAY: 22							
DAY: 8									DAY: 23							
DAY: 9									DAY: 24							
DAY: 10									DAY: 25							
DAY: 11									DAY: 26							
DAY: 12									DAY: 27							
DAY: 13									DAY: 28							
DAY: 14									DAY: 29							
DAY: 15									DAY: 30							

30 DAY
WATER
challenge

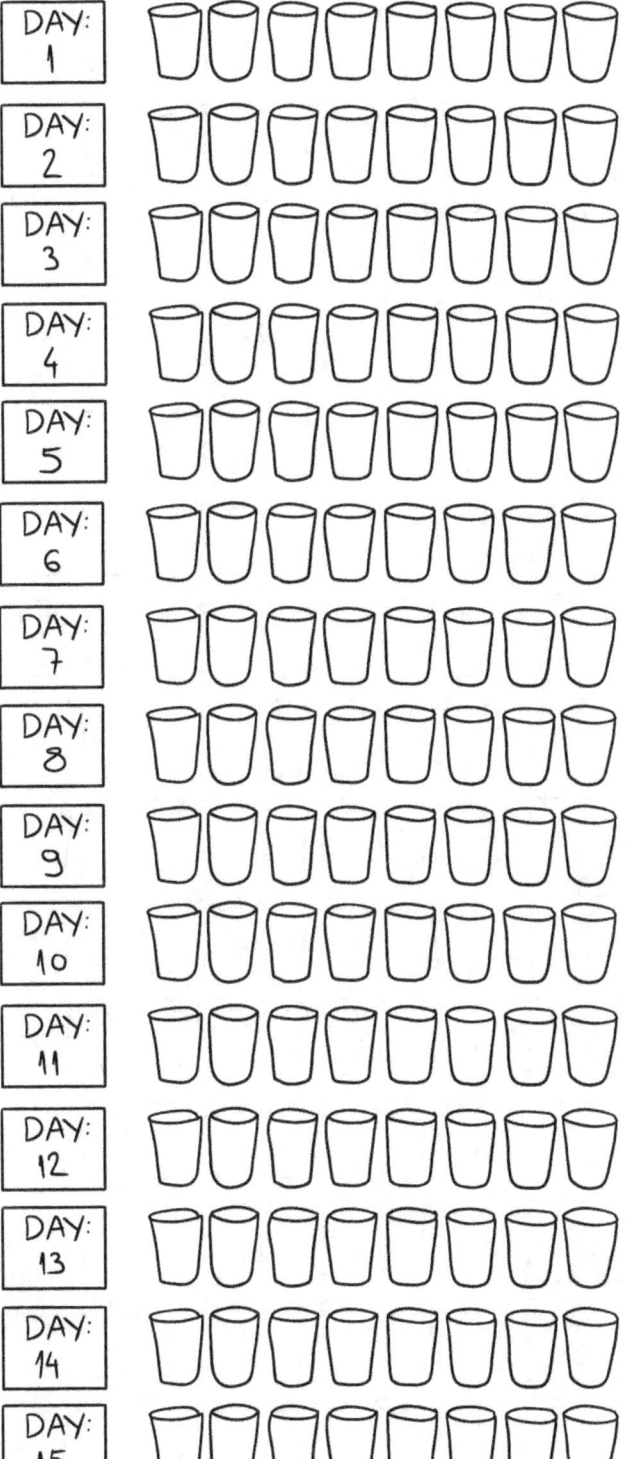

DAY: 1							
DAY: 2							
DAY: 3							
DAY: 4							
DAY: 5							
DAY: 6							
DAY: 7							
DAY: 8							
DAY: 9							
DAY: 10							
DAY: 11							
DAY: 12							
DAY: 13							
DAY: 14							
DAY: 15							

DAY: 16							
DAY: 17							
DAY: 18							
DAY: 19							
DAY: 20							
DAY: 21							
DAY: 22							
DAY: 23							
DAY: 24							
DAY: 25							
DAY: 26							
DAY: 27							
DAY: 28							
DAY: 29							
DAY: 30							

30 DAY
WATER
challenge

DAY: 1	⊔⊔⊔⊔⊔⊔⊔⊔	DAY: 16	⊔⊔⊔⊔⊔⊔⊔⊔
DAY: 2	⊔⊔⊔⊔⊔⊔⊔⊔	DAY: 17	⊔⊔⊔⊔⊔⊔⊔⊔
DAY: 3	⊔⊔⊔⊔⊔⊔⊔⊔	DAY: 18	⊔⊔⊔⊔⊔⊔⊔⊔
DAY: 4	⊔⊔⊔⊔⊔⊔⊔⊔	DAY: 19	⊔⊔⊔⊔⊔⊔⊔⊔
DAY: 5	⊔⊔⊔⊔⊔⊔⊔⊔	DAY: 20	⊔⊔⊔⊔⊔⊔⊔⊔
DAY: 6	⊔⊔⊔⊔⊔⊔⊔⊔	DAY: 21	⊔⊔⊔⊔⊔⊔⊔⊔
DAY: 7	⊔⊔⊔⊔⊔⊔⊔⊔	DAY: 22	⊔⊔⊔⊔⊔⊔⊔⊔
DAY: 8	⊔⊔⊔⊔⊔⊔⊔⊔	DAY: 23	⊔⊔⊔⊔⊔⊔⊔⊔
DAY: 9	⊔⊔⊔⊔⊔⊔⊔⊔	DAY: 24	⊔⊔⊔⊔⊔⊔⊔⊔
DAY: 10	⊔⊔⊔⊔⊔⊔⊔⊔	DAY: 25	⊔⊔⊔⊔⊔⊔⊔⊔
DAY: 11	⊔⊔⊔⊔⊔⊔⊔⊔	DAY: 26	⊔⊔⊔⊔⊔⊔⊔⊔
DAY: 12	⊔⊔⊔⊔⊔⊔⊔⊔	DAY: 27	⊔⊔⊔⊔⊔⊔⊔⊔
DAY: 13	⊔⊔⊔⊔⊔⊔⊔⊔	DAY: 28	⊔⊔⊔⊔⊔⊔⊔⊔
DAY: 14	⊔⊔⊔⊔⊔⊔⊔⊔	DAY: 29	⊔⊔⊔⊔⊔⊔⊔⊔
DAY: 15	⊔⊔⊔⊔⊔⊔⊔⊔	DAY: 30	⊔⊔⊔⊔⊔⊔⊔⊔

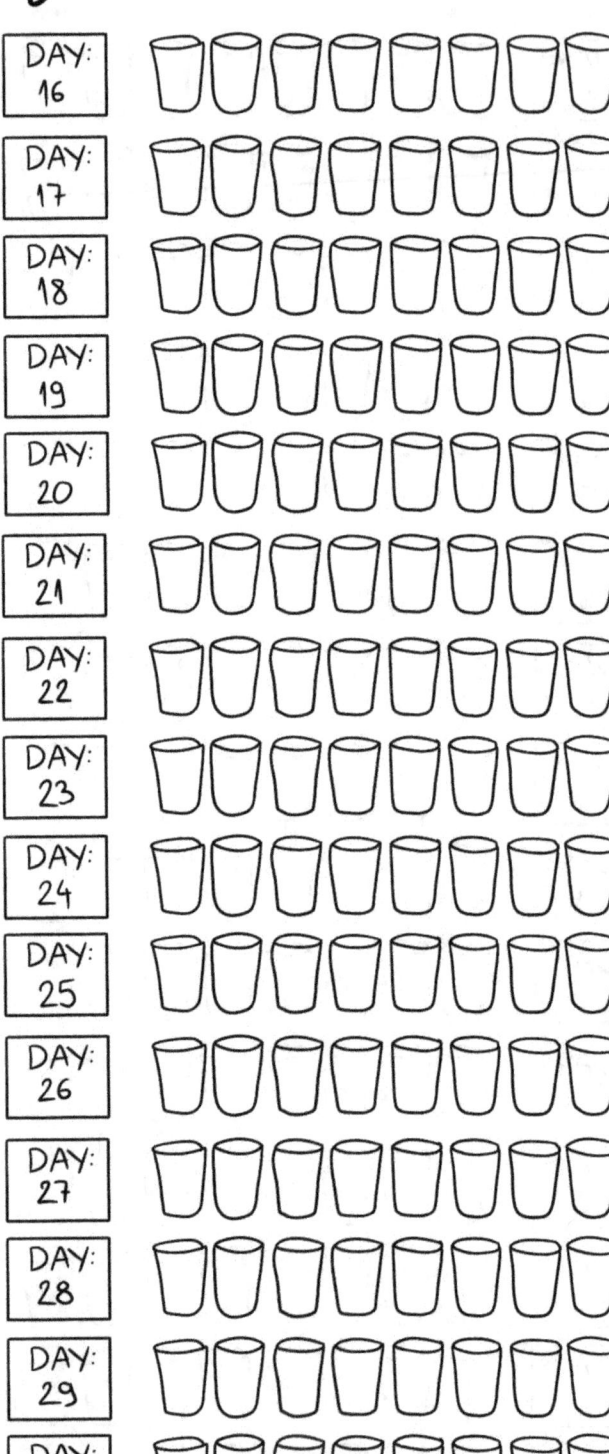

30 DAY
WATER
challenge

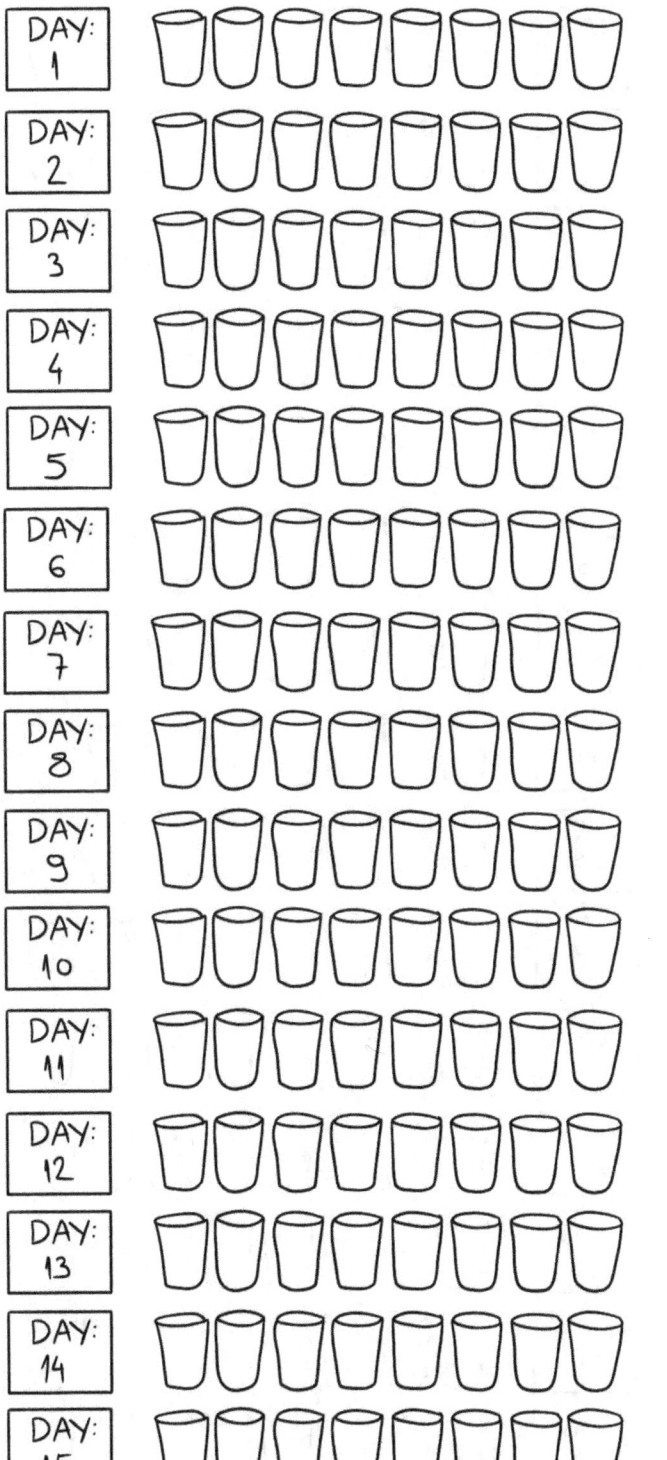

DAY: 1							
DAY: 2							
DAY: 3							
DAY: 4							
DAY: 5							
DAY: 6							
DAY: 7							
DAY: 8							
DAY: 9							
DAY: 10							
DAY: 11							
DAY: 12							
DAY: 13							
DAY: 14							
DAY: 15							

DAY: 16							
DAY: 17							
DAY: 18							
DAY: 19							
DAY: 20							
DAY: 21							
DAY: 22							
DAY: 23							
DAY: 24							
DAY: 25							
DAY: 26							
DAY: 27							
DAY: 28							
DAY: 29							
DAY: 30							

30 DAY
WATER
challenge

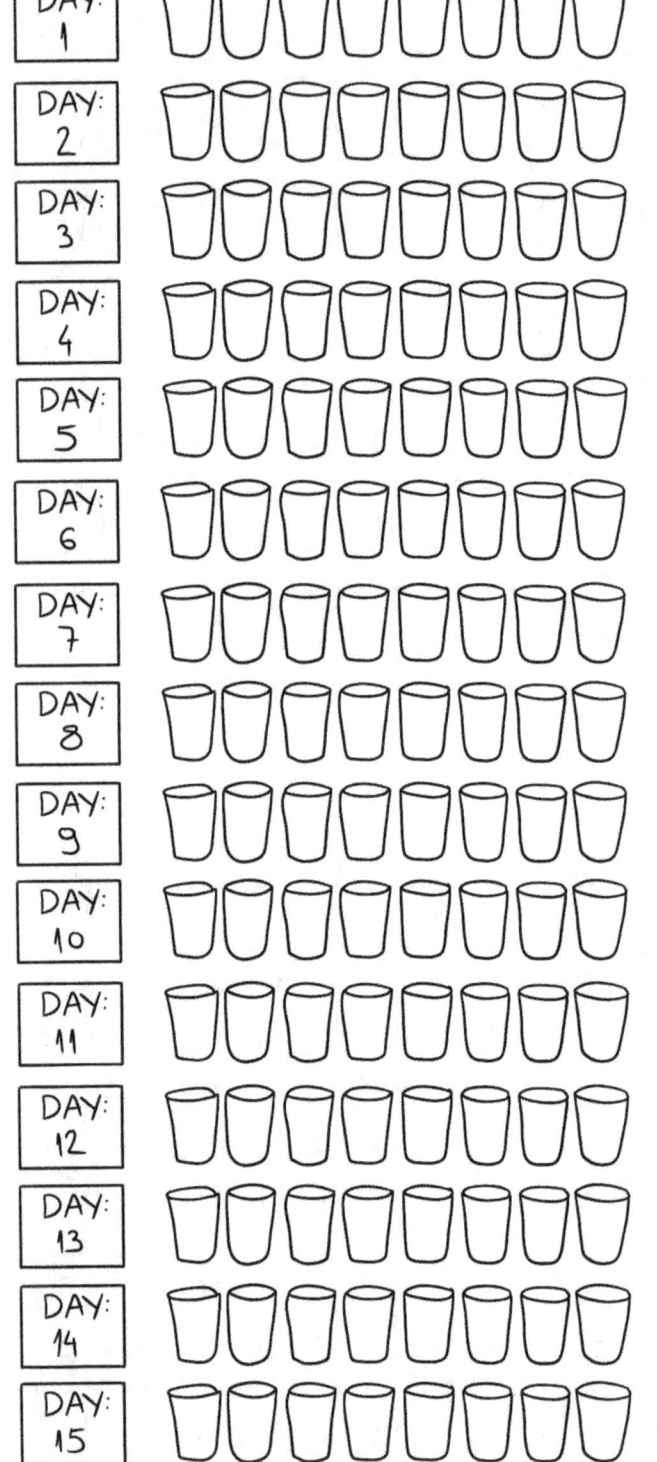

DAY: 1									DAY: 16							
DAY: 2									DAY: 17							
DAY: 3									DAY: 18							
DAY: 4									DAY: 19							
DAY: 5									DAY: 20							
DAY: 6									DAY: 21							
DAY: 7									DAY: 22							
DAY: 8									DAY: 23							
DAY: 9									DAY: 24							
DAY: 10									DAY: 25							
DAY: 11									DAY: 26							
DAY: 12									DAY: 27							
DAY: 13									DAY: 28							
DAY: 14									DAY: 29							
DAY: 15									DAY: 30							

30 DAY WATER challenge

DAY: 1								DAY: 16							
DAY: 2								DAY: 17							
DAY: 3								DAY: 18							
DAY: 4								DAY: 19							
DAY: 5								DAY: 20							
DAY: 6								DAY: 21							
DAY: 7								DAY: 22							
DAY: 8								DAY: 23							
DAY: 9								DAY: 24							
DAY: 10								DAY: 25							
DAY: 11								DAY: 26							
DAY: 12								DAY: 27							
DAY: 13								DAY: 28							
DAY: 14								DAY: 29							
DAY: 15								DAY: 30							

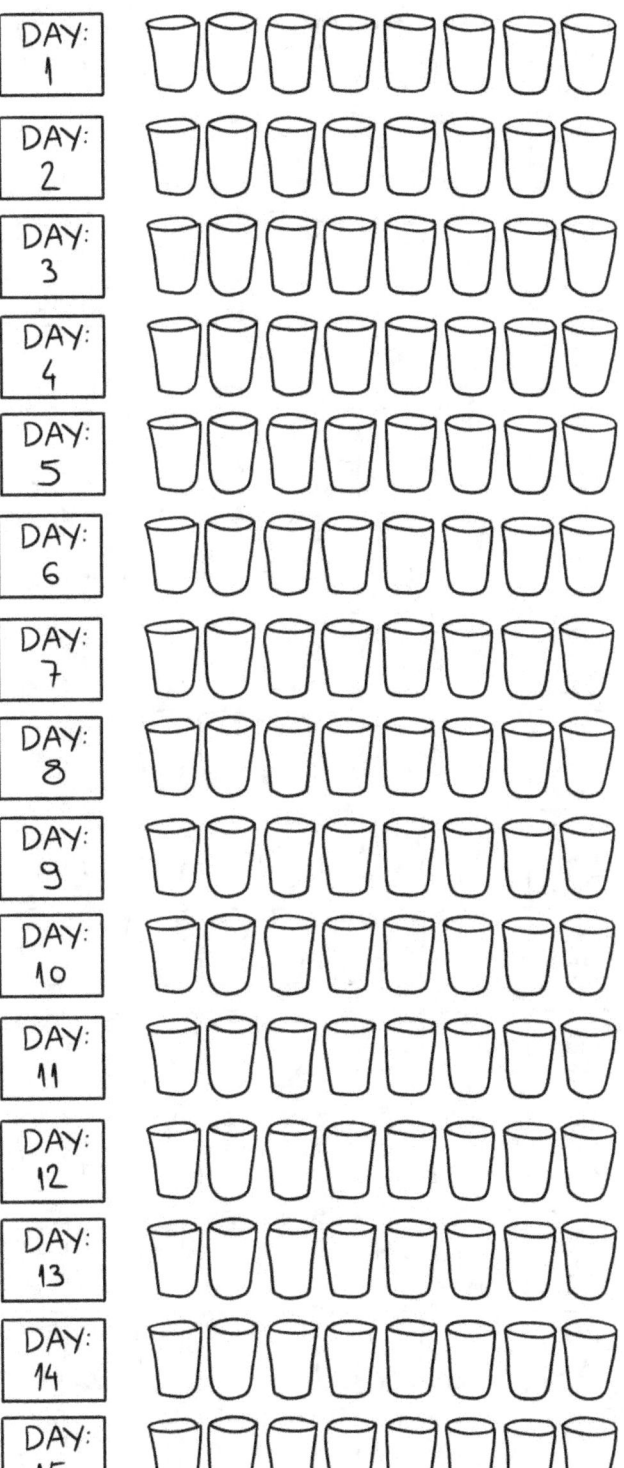

30 DAY
WATER
challenge

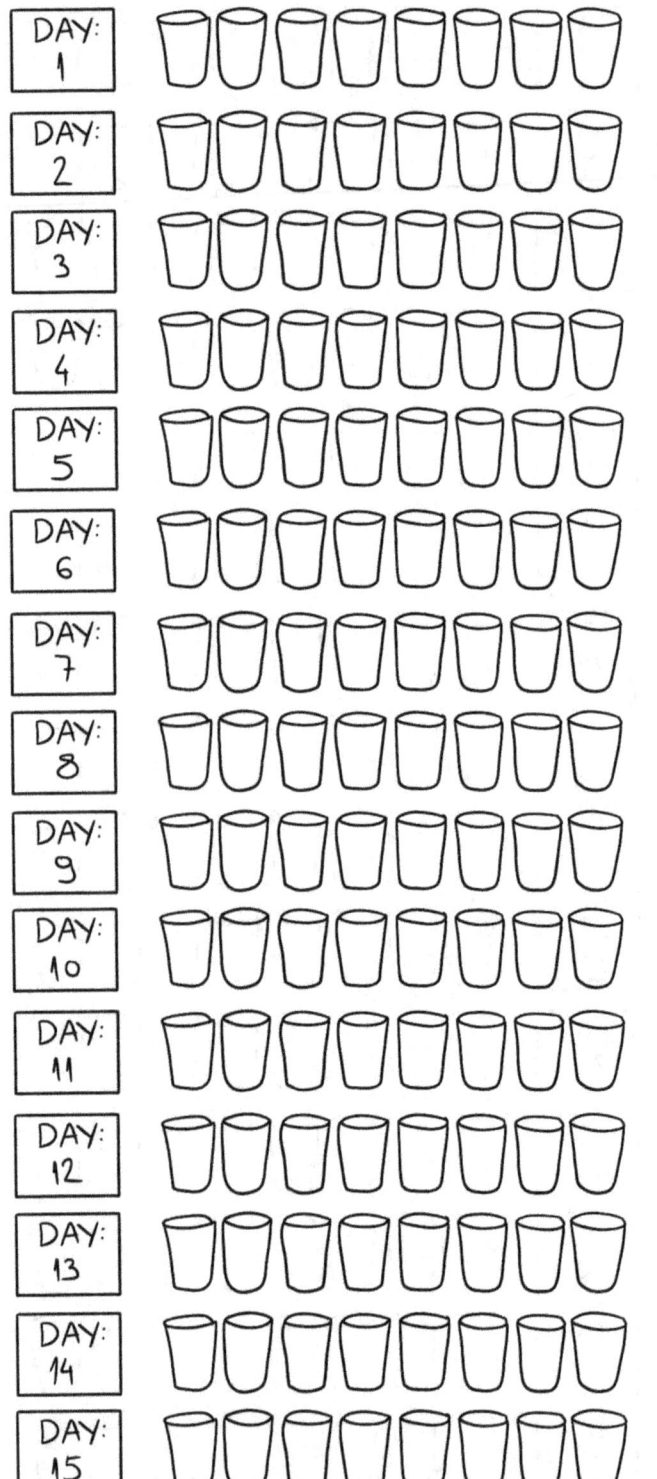

DAY: 1

DAY: 2

DAY: 3

DAY: 4

DAY: 5

DAY: 6

DAY: 7

DAY: 8

DAY: 9

DAY: 10

DAY: 11

DAY: 12

DAY: 13

DAY: 14

DAY: 15

DAY: 16

DAY: 17

DAY: 18

DAY: 19

DAY: 20

DAY: 21

DAY: 22

DAY: 23

DAY: 24

DAY: 25

DAY: 26

DAY: 27

DAY: 28

DAY: 29

DAY: 30

30 DAY WATER challenge

DAY: 1	⊔ ⊔ ⊔ ⊔ ⊔ ⊔ ⊔ ⊔	DAY: 16	⊔ ⊔ ⊔ ⊔ ⊔ ⊔ ⊔ ⊔
DAY: 2	⊔ ⊔ ⊔ ⊔ ⊔ ⊔ ⊔ ⊔	DAY: 17	⊔ ⊔ ⊔ ⊔ ⊔ ⊔ ⊔ ⊔
DAY: 3	⊔ ⊔ ⊔ ⊔ ⊔ ⊔ ⊔ ⊔	DAY: 18	⊔ ⊔ ⊔ ⊔ ⊔ ⊔ ⊔ ⊔
DAY: 4	⊔ ⊔ ⊔ ⊔ ⊔ ⊔ ⊔ ⊔	DAY: 19	⊔ ⊔ ⊔ ⊔ ⊔ ⊔ ⊔ ⊔
DAY: 5	⊔ ⊔ ⊔ ⊔ ⊔ ⊔ ⊔ ⊔	DAY: 20	⊔ ⊔ ⊔ ⊔ ⊔ ⊔ ⊔ ⊔
DAY: 6	⊔ ⊔ ⊔ ⊔ ⊔ ⊔ ⊔ ⊔	DAY: 21	⊔ ⊔ ⊔ ⊔ ⊔ ⊔ ⊔ ⊔
DAY: 7	⊔ ⊔ ⊔ ⊔ ⊔ ⊔ ⊔ ⊔	DAY: 22	⊔ ⊔ ⊔ ⊔ ⊔ ⊔ ⊔ ⊔
DAY: 8	⊔ ⊔ ⊔ ⊔ ⊔ ⊔ ⊔ ⊔	DAY: 23	⊔ ⊔ ⊔ ⊔ ⊔ ⊔ ⊔ ⊔
DAY: 9	⊔ ⊔ ⊔ ⊔ ⊔ ⊔ ⊔ ⊔	DAY: 24	⊔ ⊔ ⊔ ⊔ ⊔ ⊔ ⊔ ⊔
DAY: 10	⊔ ⊔ ⊔ ⊔ ⊔ ⊔ ⊔ ⊔	DAY: 25	⊔ ⊔ ⊔ ⊔ ⊔ ⊔ ⊔ ⊔
DAY: 11	⊔ ⊔ ⊔ ⊔ ⊔ ⊔ ⊔ ⊔	DAY: 26	⊔ ⊔ ⊔ ⊔ ⊔ ⊔ ⊔ ⊔
DAY: 12	⊔ ⊔ ⊔ ⊔ ⊔ ⊔ ⊔ ⊔	DAY: 27	⊔ ⊔ ⊔ ⊔ ⊔ ⊔ ⊔ ⊔
DAY: 13	⊔ ⊔ ⊔ ⊔ ⊔ ⊔ ⊔ ⊔	DAY: 28	⊔ ⊔ ⊔ ⊔ ⊔ ⊔ ⊔ ⊔
DAY: 14	⊔ ⊔ ⊔ ⊔ ⊔ ⊔ ⊔ ⊔	DAY: 29	⊔ ⊔ ⊔ ⊔ ⊔ ⊔ ⊔ ⊔
DAY: 15	⊔ ⊔ ⊔ ⊔ ⊔ ⊔ ⊔ ⊔	DAY: 30	⊔ ⊔ ⊔ ⊔ ⊔ ⊔ ⊔ ⊔

30 DAY
WATER
challenge

DAY: 1								
DAY: 2								
DAY: 3								
DAY: 4								
DAY: 5								
DAY: 6								
DAY: 7								
DAY: 8								
DAY: 9								
DAY: 10								
DAY: 11								
DAY: 12								
DAY: 13								
DAY: 14								
DAY: 15								

DAY: 16								
DAY: 17								
DAY: 18								
DAY: 19								
DAY: 20								
DAY: 21								
DAY: 22								
DAY: 23								
DAY: 24								
DAY: 25								
DAY: 26								
DAY: 27								
DAY: 28								
DAY: 29								
DAY: 30								

30 DAY
WATER
challenge

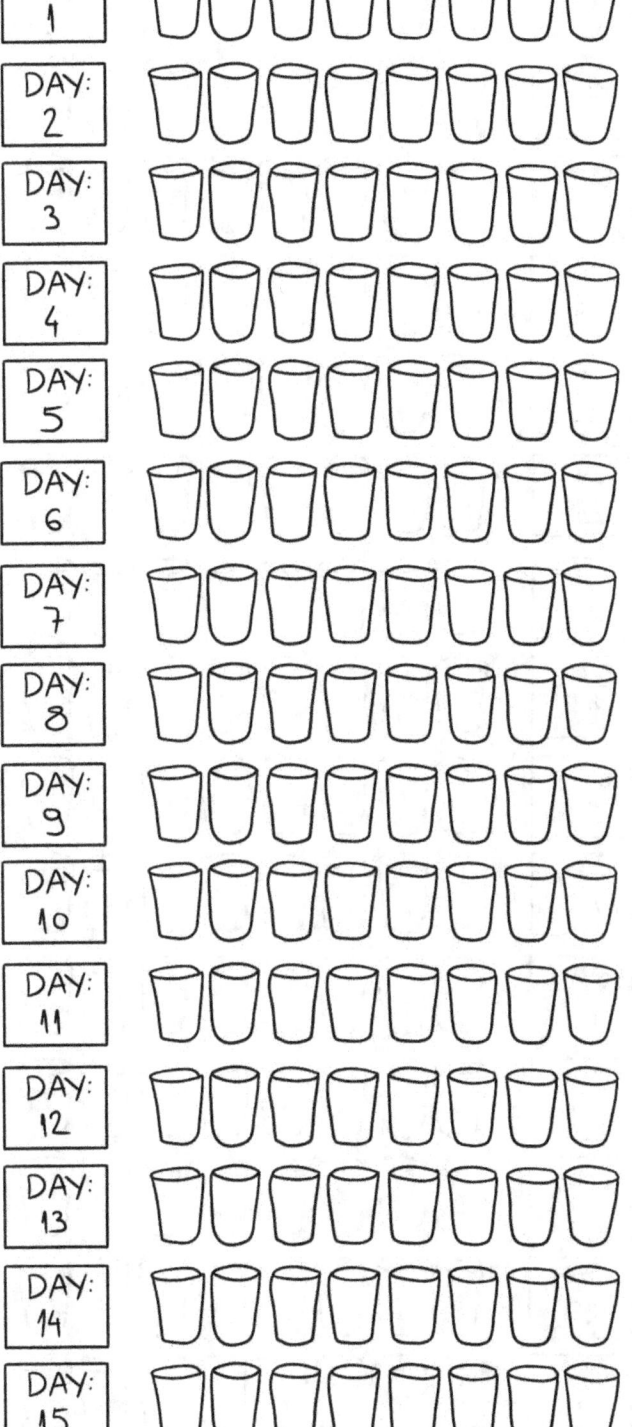

DAY: 1								
DAY: 2								
DAY: 3								
DAY: 4								
DAY: 5								
DAY: 6								
DAY: 7								
DAY: 8								
DAY: 9								
DAY: 10								
DAY: 11								
DAY: 12								
DAY: 13								
DAY: 14								
DAY: 15								

DAY: 16								
DAY: 17								
DAY: 18								
DAY: 19								
DAY: 20								
DAY: 21								
DAY: 22								
DAY: 23								
DAY: 24								
DAY: 25								
DAY: 26								
DAY: 27								
DAY: 28								
DAY: 29								
DAY: 30								

30 DAY
WATER
challenge

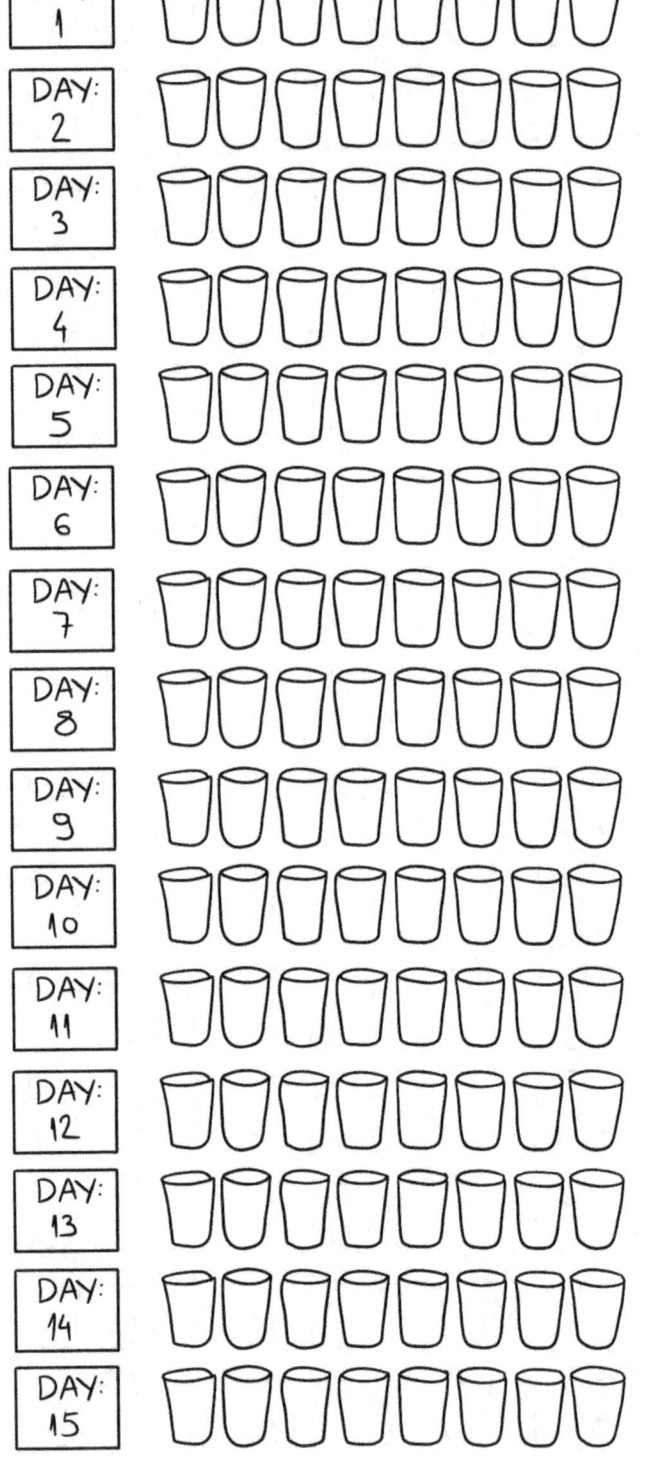
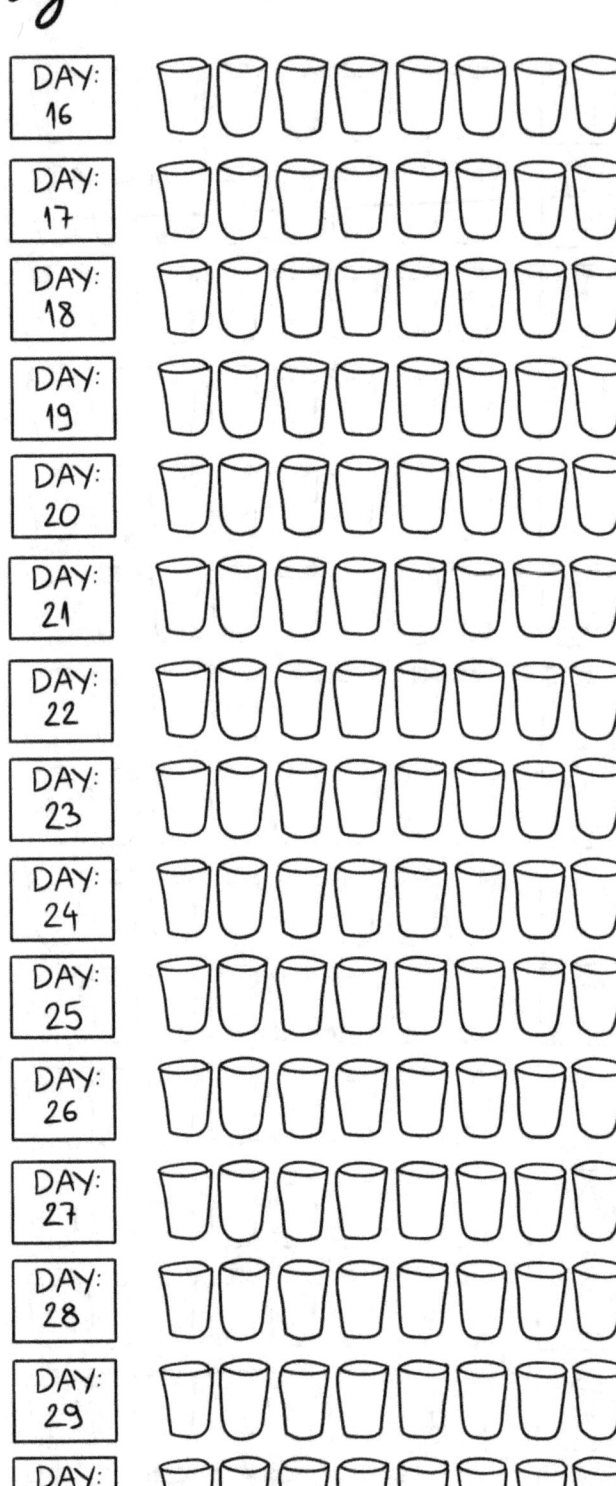

DAY: 1	DAY: 16
DAY: 2	DAY: 17
DAY: 3	DAY: 18
DAY: 4	DAY: 19
DAY: 5	DAY: 20
DAY: 6	DAY: 21
DAY: 7	DAY: 22
DAY: 8	DAY: 23
DAY: 9	DAY: 24
DAY: 10	DAY: 25
DAY: 11	DAY: 26
DAY: 12	DAY: 27
DAY: 13	DAY: 28
DAY: 14	DAY: 29
DAY: 15	DAY: 30

30 DAY
WATER
challenge

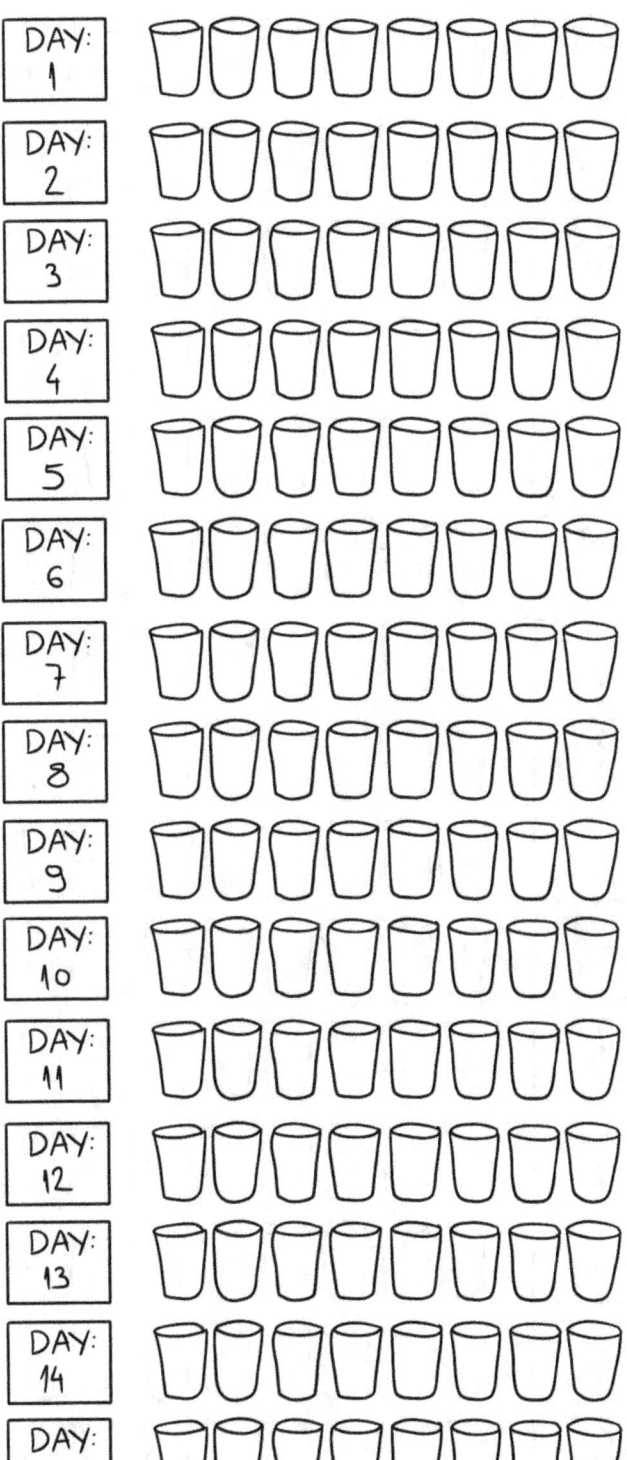

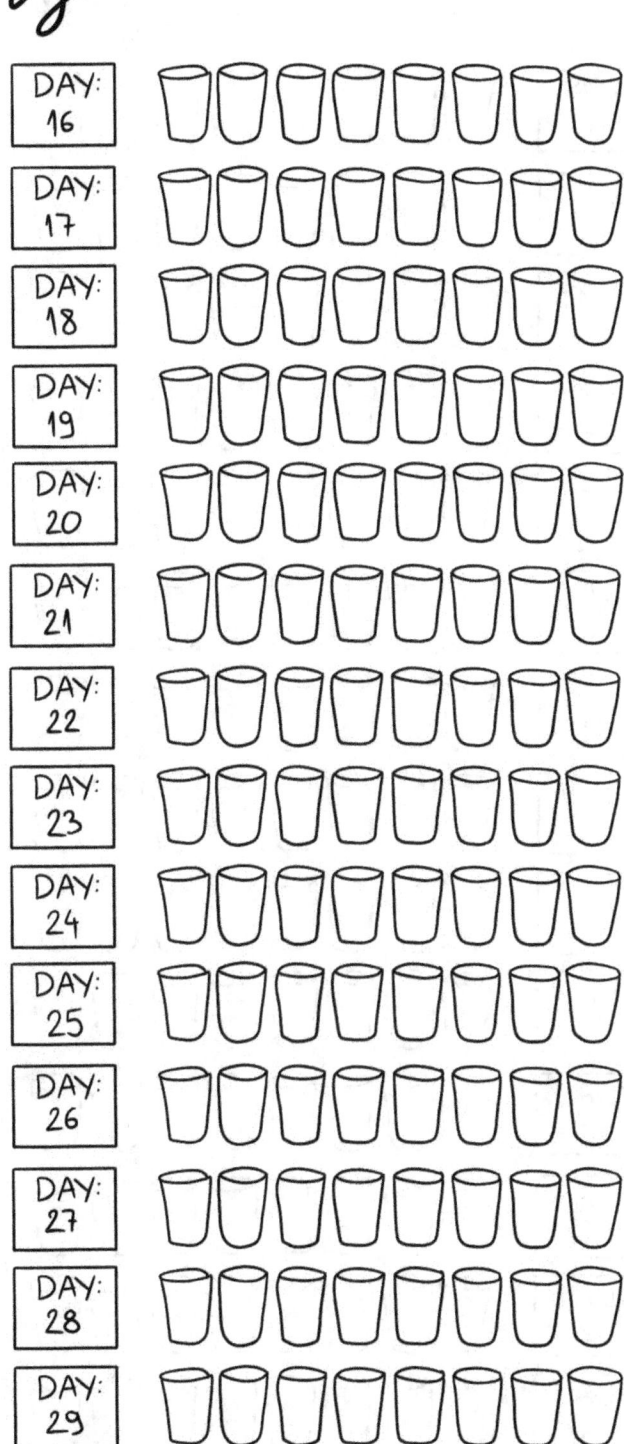

30 DAY WATER challenge

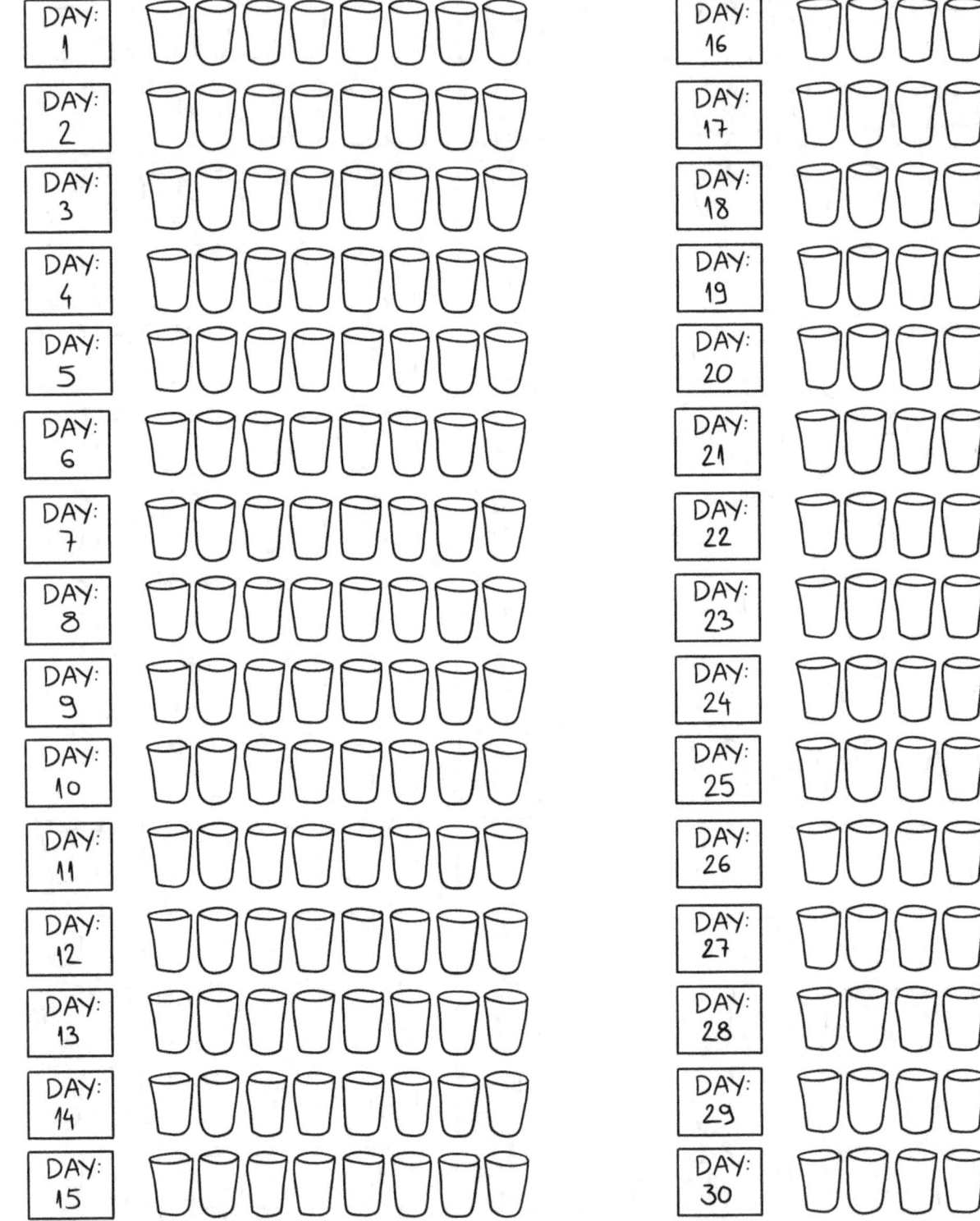

30 DAY WATER challenge

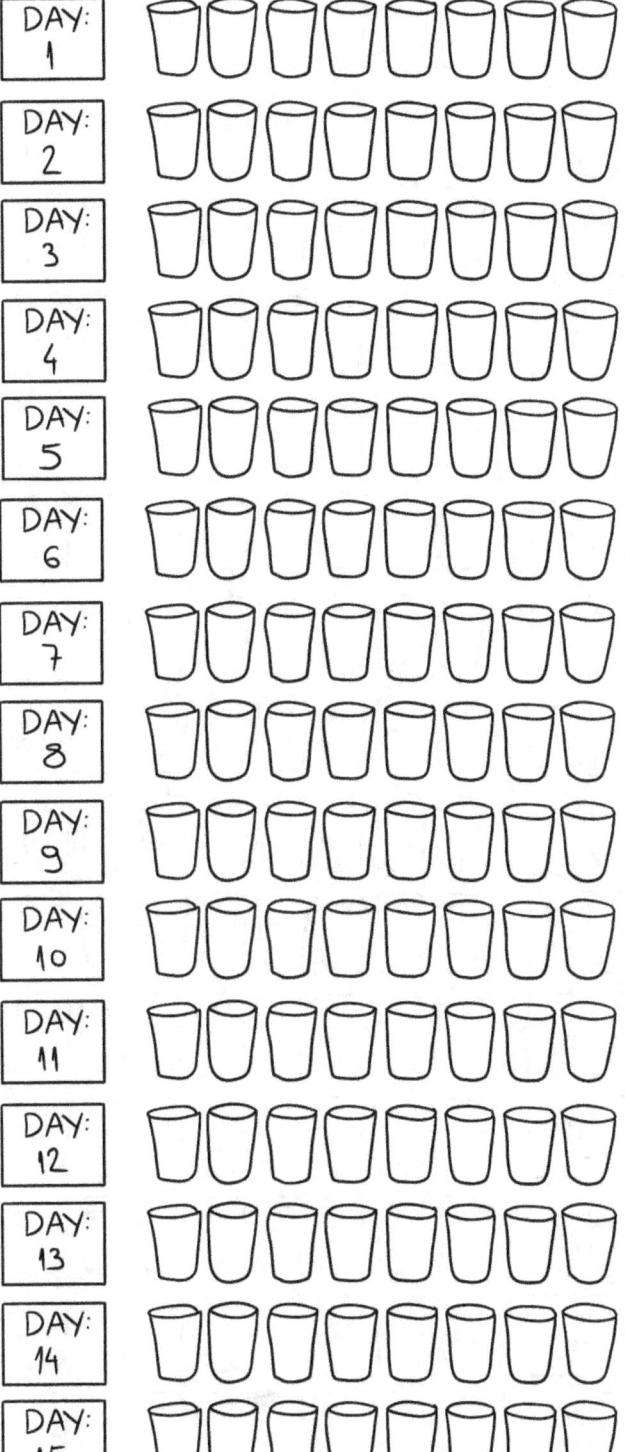

DAY: 1								
DAY: 2								
DAY: 3								
DAY: 4								
DAY: 5								
DAY: 6								
DAY: 7								
DAY: 8								
DAY: 9								
DAY: 10								
DAY: 11								
DAY: 12								
DAY: 13								
DAY: 14								
DAY: 15								

DAY: 16								
DAY: 17								
DAY: 18								
DAY: 19								
DAY: 20								
DAY: 21								
DAY: 22								
DAY: 23								
DAY: 24								
DAY: 25								
DAY: 26								
DAY: 27								
DAY: 28								
DAY: 29								
DAY: 30								

30 DAY
WATER
challenge

| DAY: 1 |
| DAY: 2 |
| DAY: 3 |
| DAY: 4 |
| DAY: 5 |
| DAY: 6 |
| DAY: 7 |
| DAY: 8 |
| DAY: 9 |
| DAY: 10 |
| DAY: 11 |
| DAY: 12 |
| DAY: 13 |
| DAY: 14 |
| DAY: 15 |

| DAY: 16 |
| DAY: 17 |
| DAY: 18 |
| DAY: 19 |
| DAY: 20 |
| DAY: 21 |
| DAY: 22 |
| DAY: 23 |
| DAY: 24 |
| DAY: 25 |
| DAY: 26 |
| DAY: 27 |
| DAY: 28 |
| DAY: 29 |
| DAY: 30 |

30 DAY
WATER
challenge

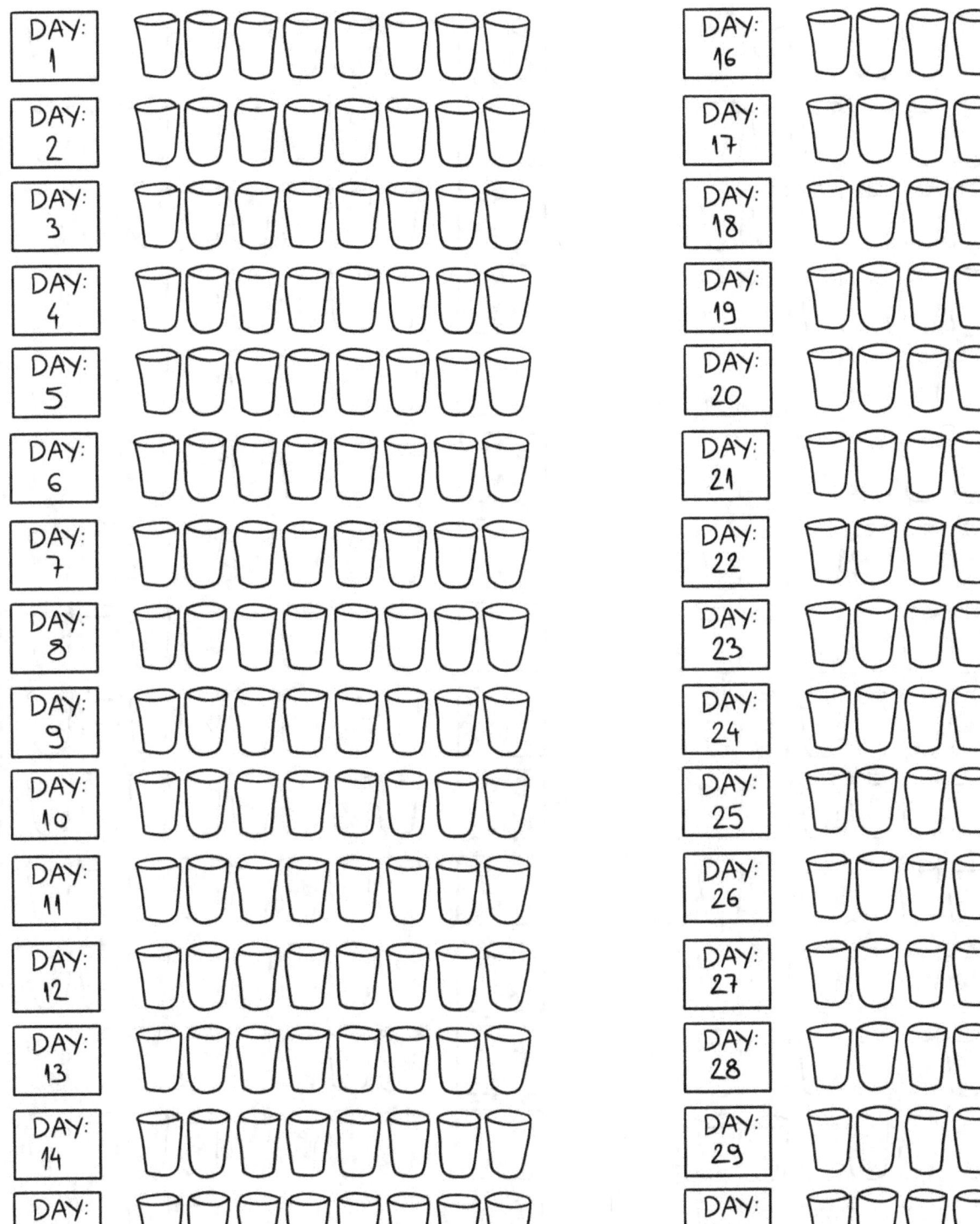

30 DAY
WATER
challenge

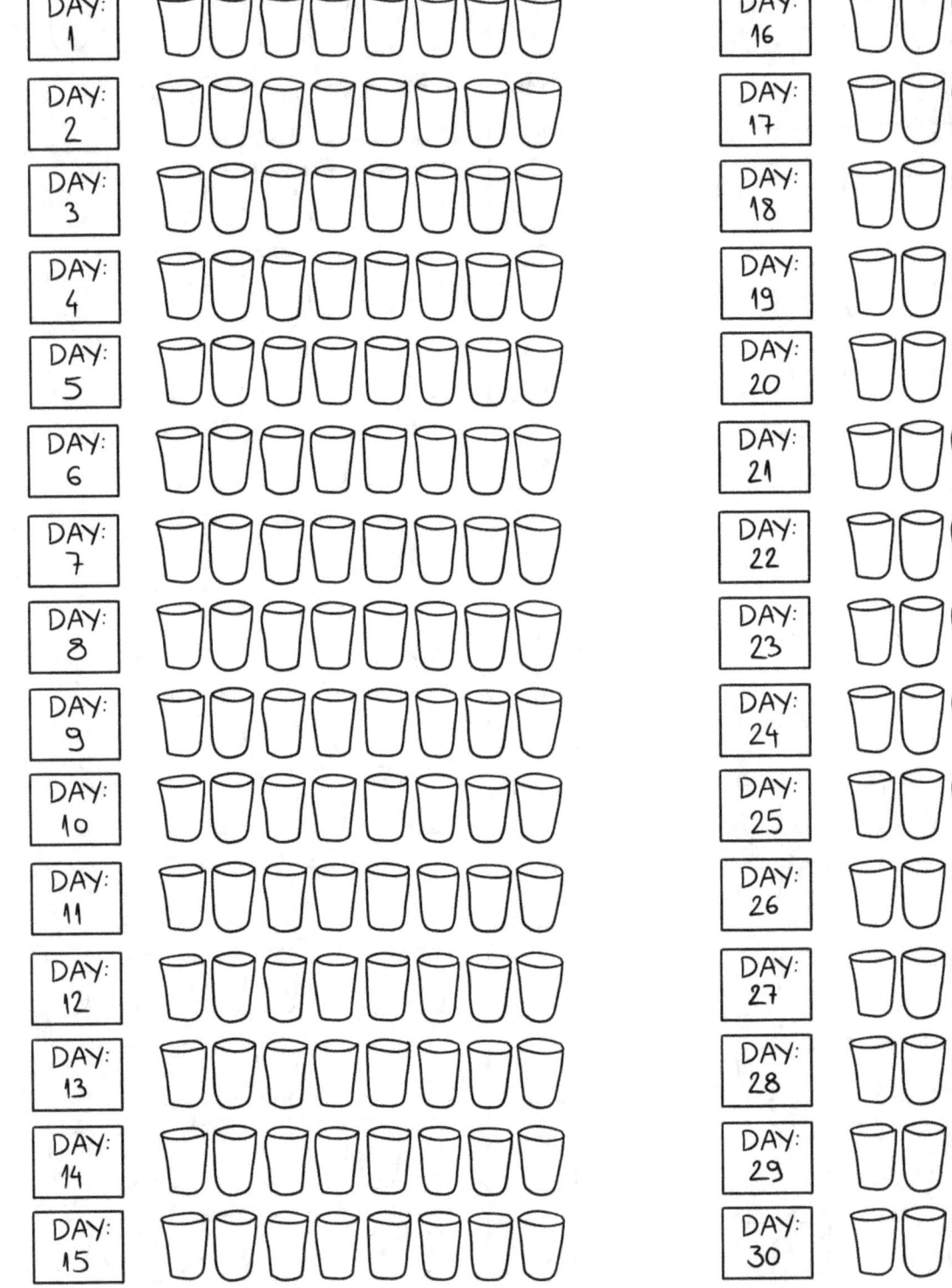

30 DAY
WATER
challenge

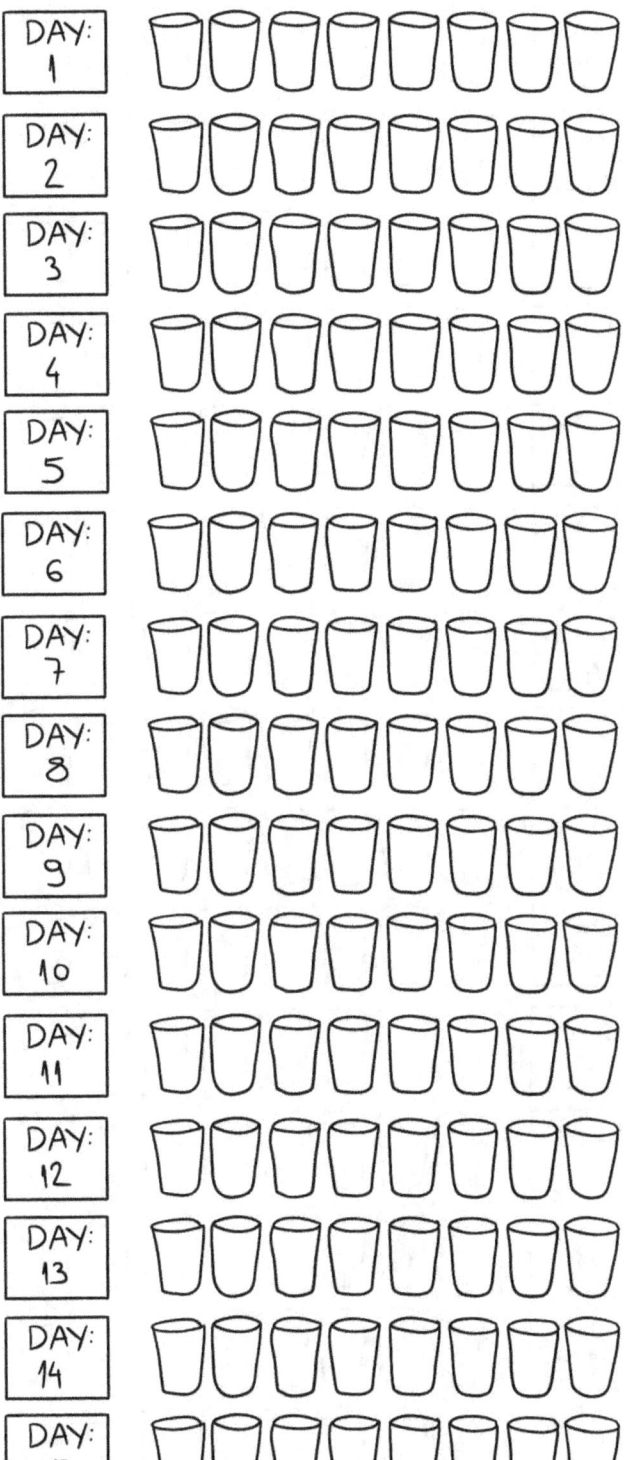
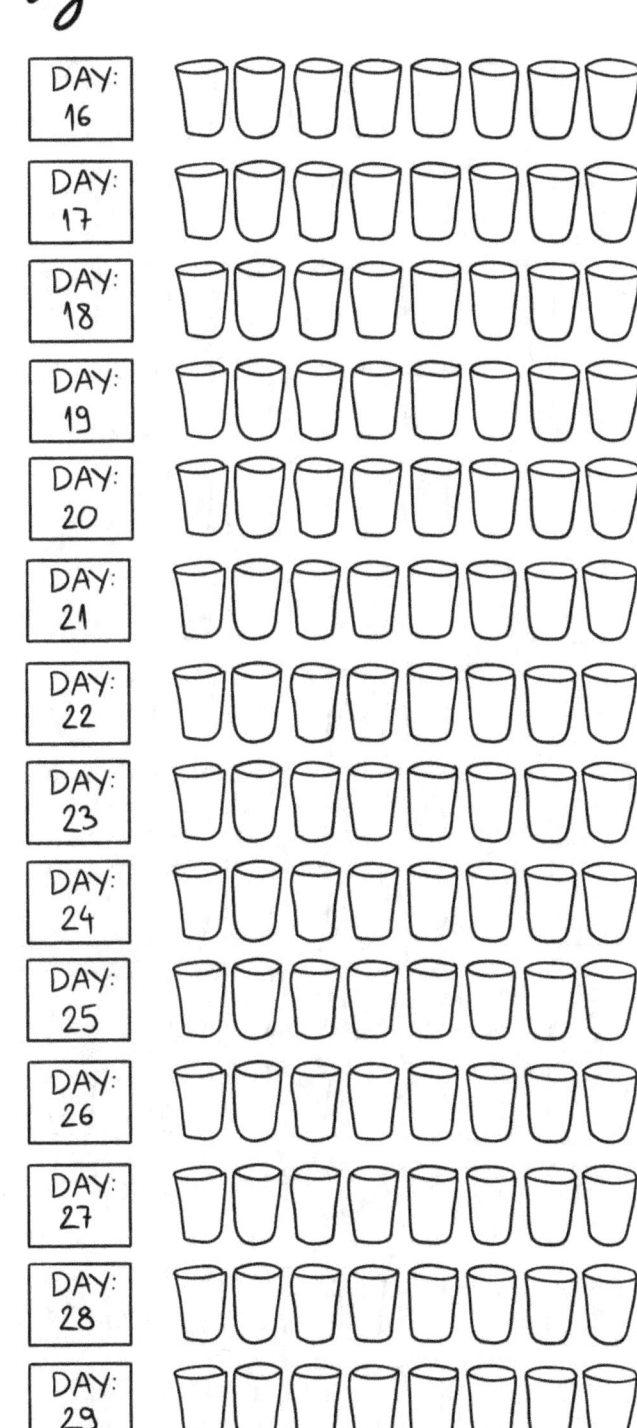

30 DAY
WATER
challenge

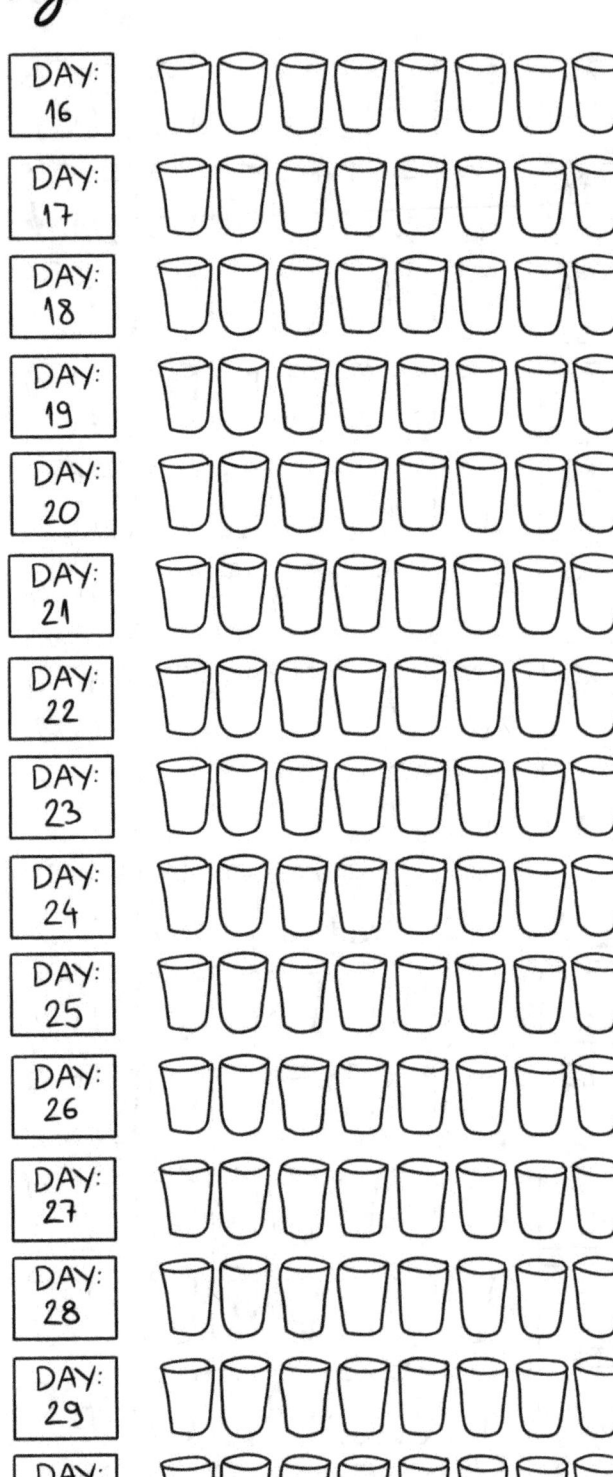

DAY: 1							
DAY: 2							
DAY: 3							
DAY: 4							
DAY: 5							
DAY: 6							
DAY: 7							
DAY: 8							
DAY: 9							
DAY: 10							
DAY: 11							
DAY: 12							
DAY: 13							
DAY: 14							
DAY: 15							

DAY: 16
DAY: 17
DAY: 18
DAY: 19
DAY: 20
DAY: 21
DAY: 22
DAY: 23
DAY: 24
DAY: 25
DAY: 26
DAY: 27
DAY: 28
DAY: 29
DAY: 30

30 DAY
WATER
challenge

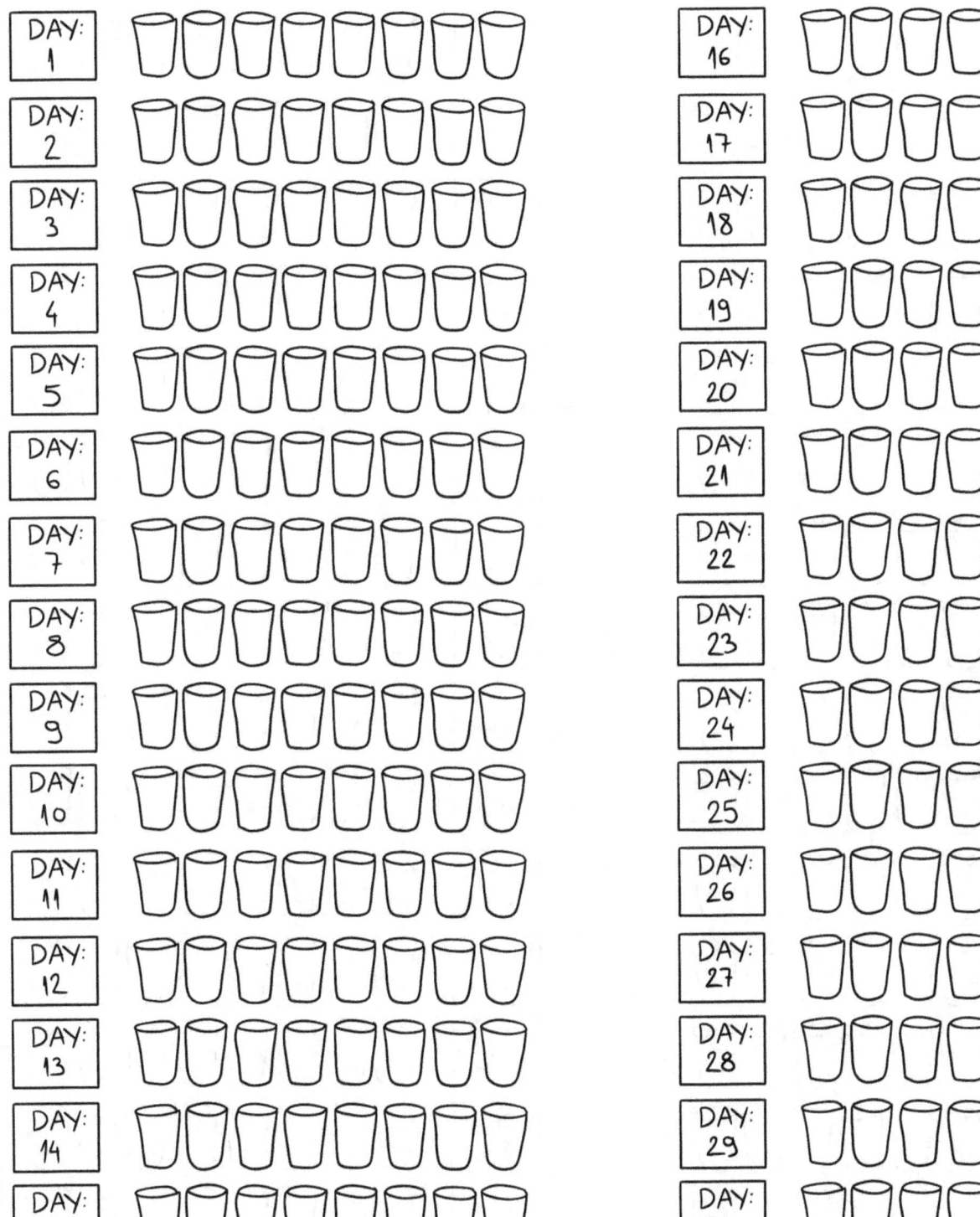

30 DAY
WATER
challenge

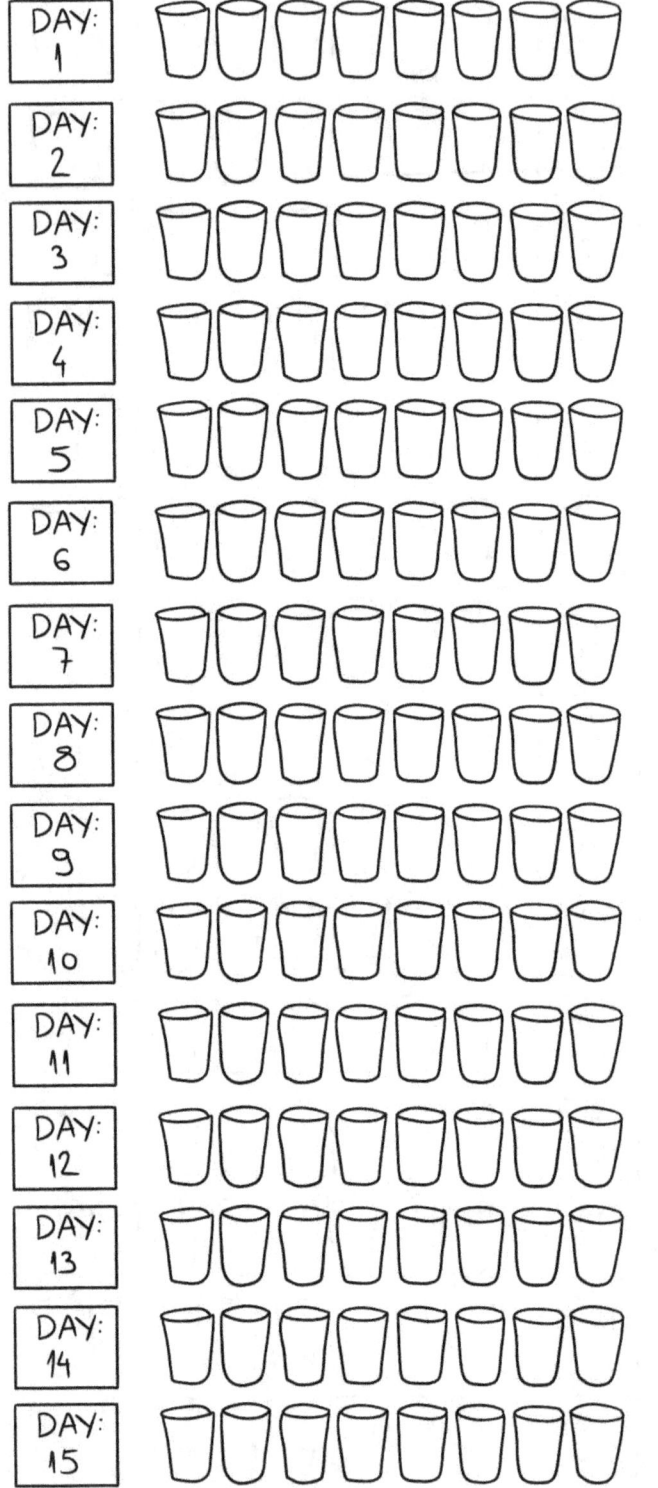
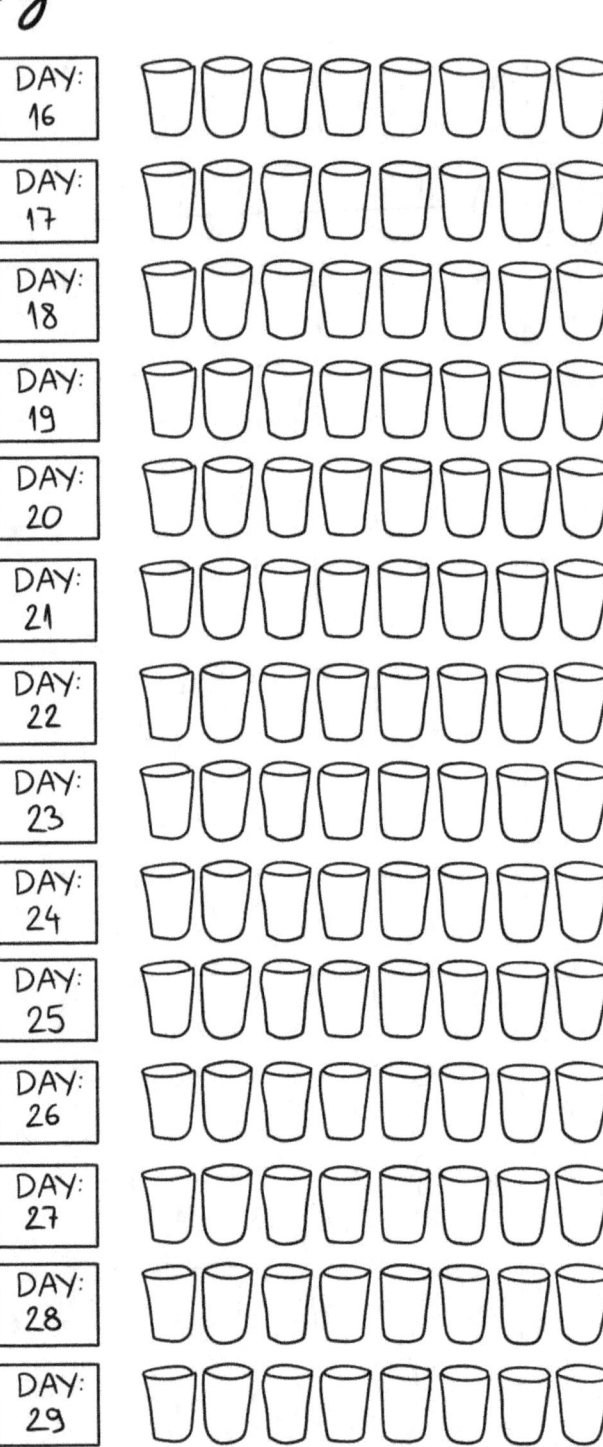

30 DAY
WATER
challenge

DAY: 1	☐☐☐☐☐☐☐☐	DAY: 16	☐☐☐☐☐☐☐☐
DAY: 2	☐☐☐☐☐☐☐☐	DAY: 17	☐☐☐☐☐☐☐☐
DAY: 3	☐☐☐☐☐☐☐☐	DAY: 18	☐☐☐☐☐☐☐☐
DAY: 4	☐☐☐☐☐☐☐☐	DAY: 19	☐☐☐☐☐☐☐☐
DAY: 5	☐☐☐☐☐☐☐☐	DAY: 20	☐☐☐☐☐☐☐☐
DAY: 6	☐☐☐☐☐☐☐☐	DAY: 21	☐☐☐☐☐☐☐☐
DAY: 7	☐☐☐☐☐☐☐☐	DAY: 22	☐☐☐☐☐☐☐☐
DAY: 8	☐☐☐☐☐☐☐☐	DAY: 23	☐☐☐☐☐☐☐☐
DAY: 9	☐☐☐☐☐☐☐☐	DAY: 24	☐☐☐☐☐☐☐☐
DAY: 10	☐☐☐☐☐☐☐☐	DAY: 25	☐☐☐☐☐☐☐☐
DAY: 11	☐☐☐☐☐☐☐☐	DAY: 26	☐☐☐☐☐☐☐☐
DAY: 12	☐☐☐☐☐☐☐☐	DAY: 27	☐☐☐☐☐☐☐☐
DAY: 13	☐☐☐☐☐☐☐☐	DAY: 28	☐☐☐☐☐☐☐☐
DAY: 14	☐☐☐☐☐☐☐☐	DAY: 29	☐☐☐☐☐☐☐☐
DAY: 15	☐☐☐☐☐☐☐☐	DAY: 30	☐☐☐☐☐☐☐☐

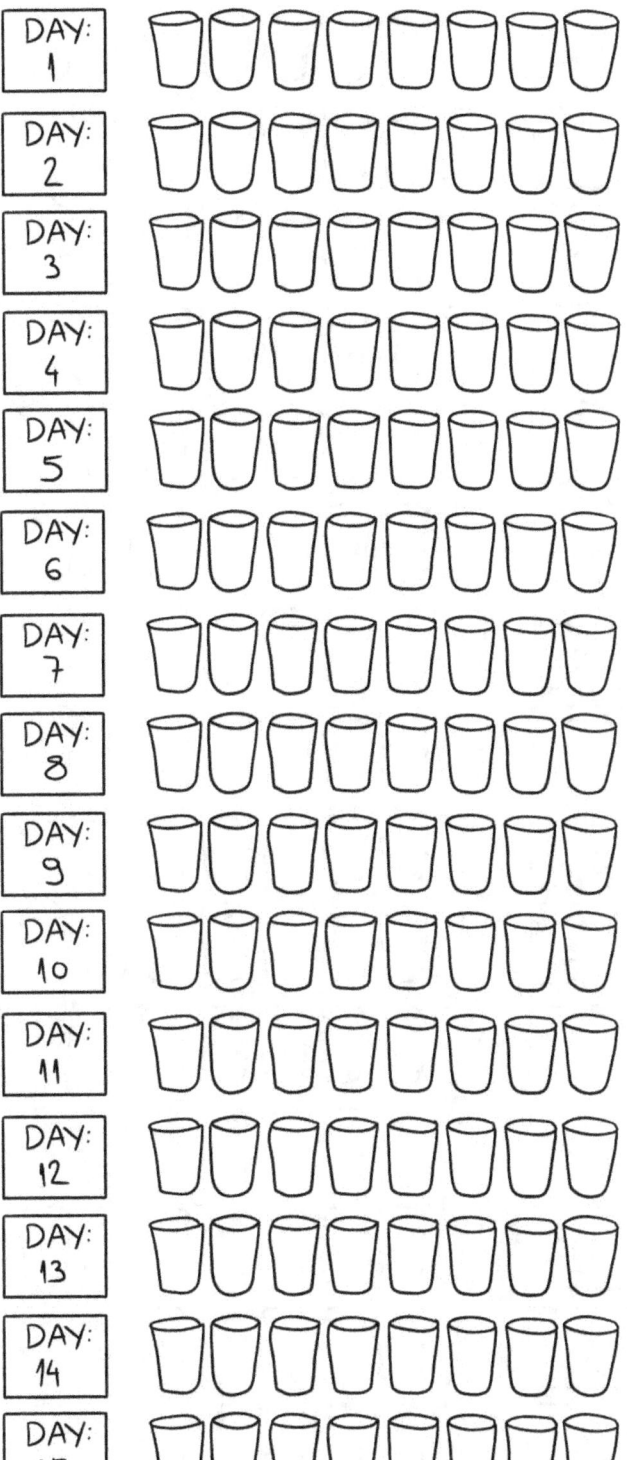

30 DAY
WATER
challenge

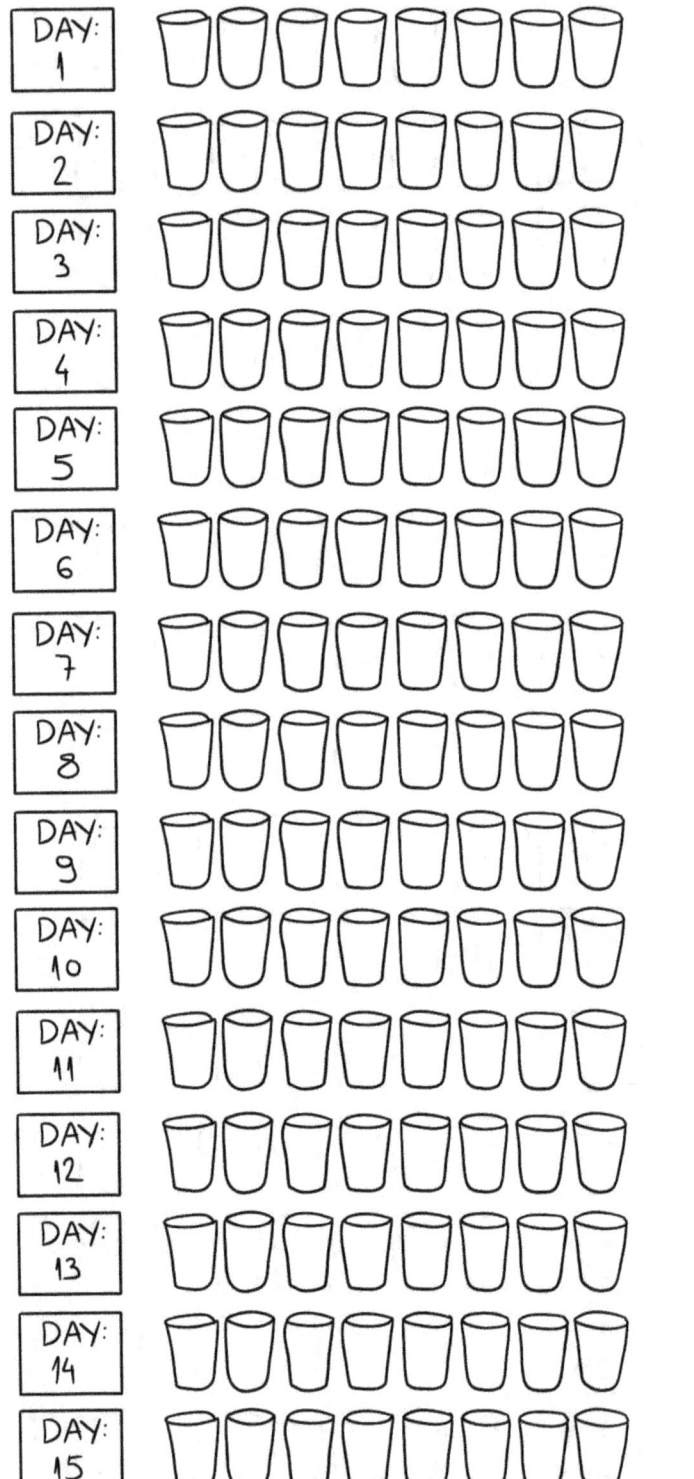

DAY: 1							
DAY: 2							
DAY: 3							
DAY: 4							
DAY: 5							
DAY: 6							
DAY: 7							
DAY: 8							
DAY: 9							
DAY: 10							
DAY: 11							
DAY: 12							
DAY: 13							
DAY: 14							
DAY: 15							

DAY: 16							
DAY: 17							
DAY: 18							
DAY: 19							
DAY: 20							
DAY: 21							
DAY: 22							
DAY: 23							
DAY: 24							
DAY: 25							
DAY: 26							
DAY: 27							
DAY: 28							
DAY: 29							
DAY: 30							

30 DAY
WATER
challenge

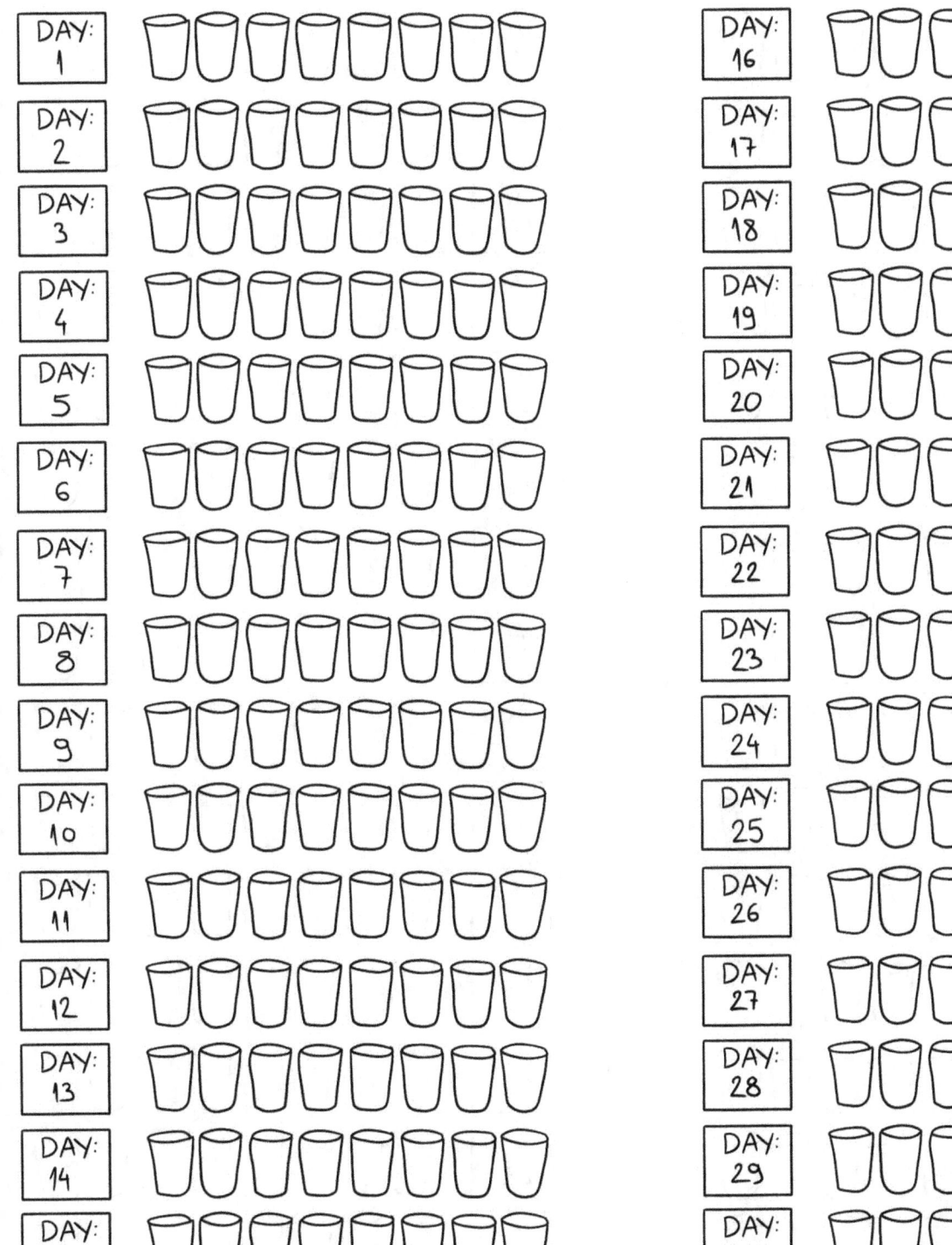

DAY: 1		DAY: 16	
DAY: 2		DAY: 17	
DAY: 3		DAY: 18	
DAY: 4		DAY: 19	
DAY: 5		DAY: 20	
DAY: 6		DAY: 21	
DAY: 7		DAY: 22	
DAY: 8		DAY: 23	
DAY: 9		DAY: 24	
DAY: 10		DAY: 25	
DAY: 11		DAY: 26	
DAY: 12		DAY: 27	
DAY: 13		DAY: 28	
DAY: 14		DAY: 29	
DAY: 15		DAY: 30	

30 DAY
WATER
challenge

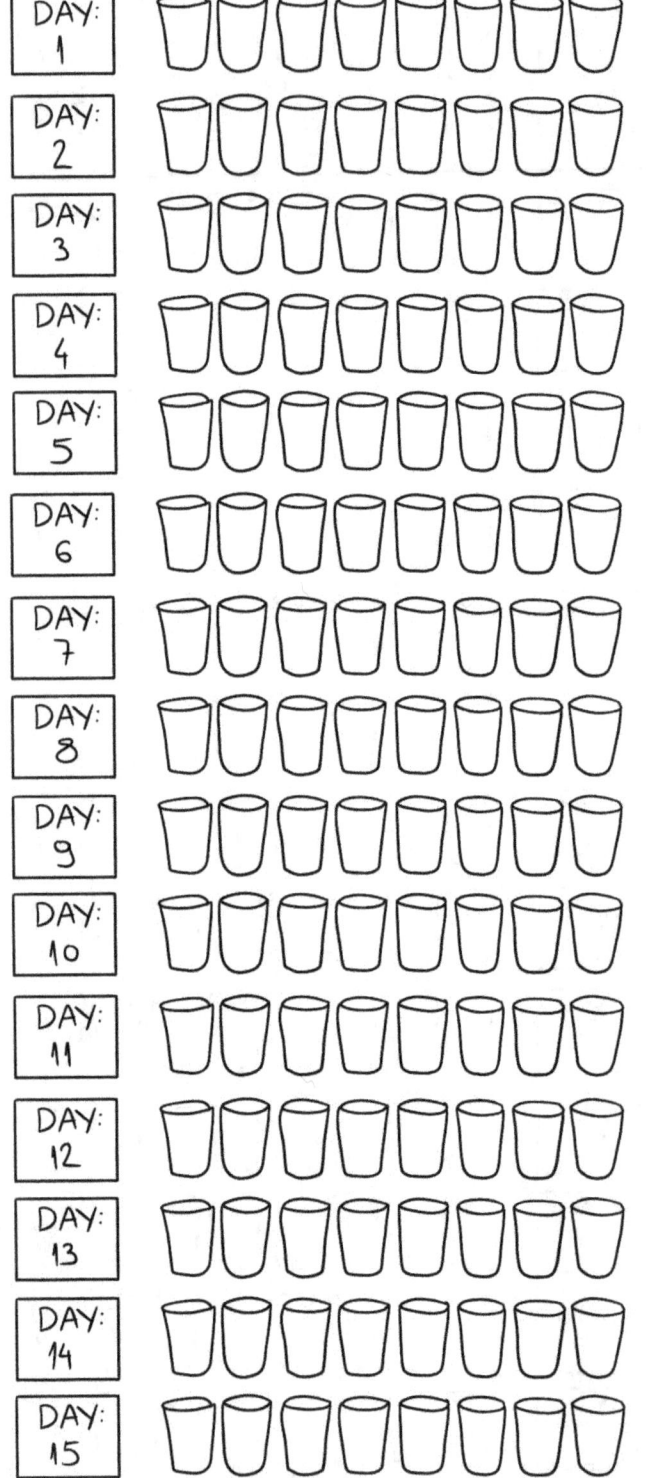

DAY: 1	DAY: 16
DAY: 2	DAY: 17
DAY: 3	DAY: 18
DAY: 4	DAY: 19
DAY: 5	DAY: 20
DAY: 6	DAY: 21
DAY: 7	DAY: 22
DAY: 8	DAY: 23
DAY: 9	DAY: 24
DAY: 10	DAY: 25
DAY: 11	DAY: 26
DAY: 12	DAY: 27
DAY: 13	DAY: 28
DAY: 14	DAY: 29
DAY: 15	DAY: 30

30 DAY
WATER
challenge

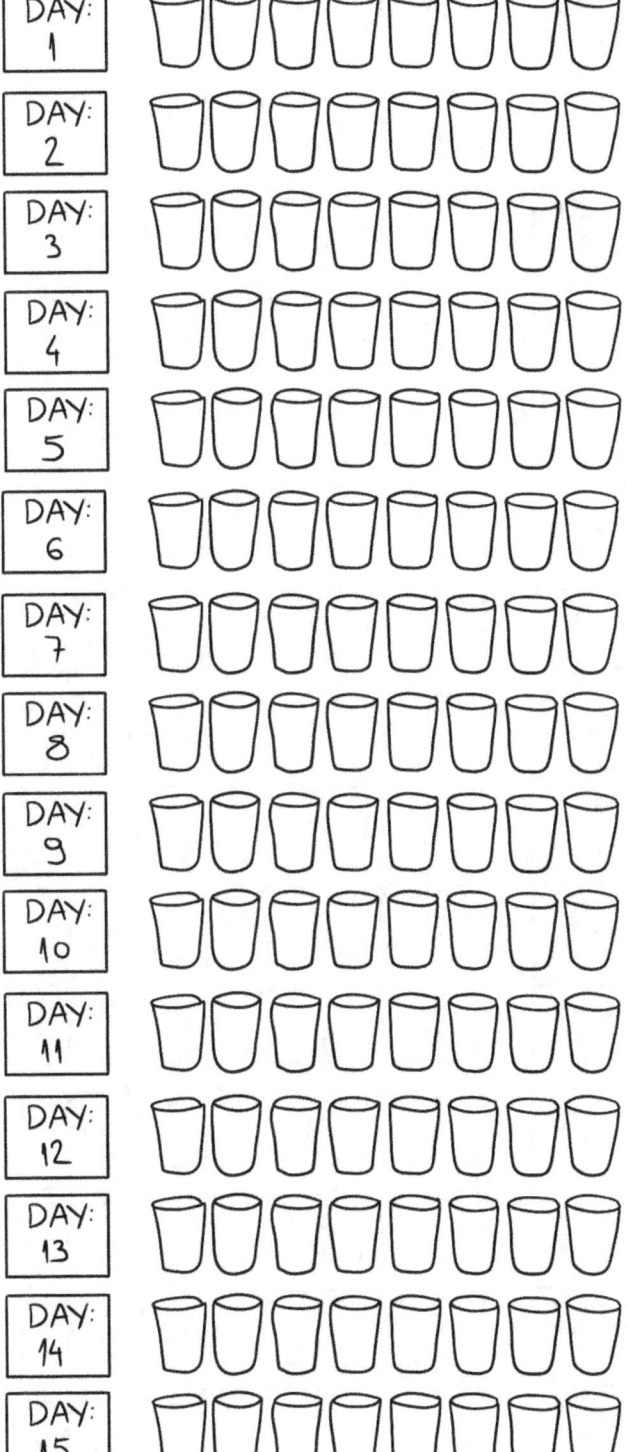

DAY: 1	🥛🥛🥛🥛🥛🥛🥛🥛
DAY: 2	🥛🥛🥛🥛🥛🥛🥛🥛
DAY: 3	🥛🥛🥛🥛🥛🥛🥛🥛
DAY: 4	🥛🥛🥛🥛🥛🥛🥛🥛
DAY: 5	🥛🥛🥛🥛🥛🥛🥛🥛
DAY: 6	🥛🥛🥛🥛🥛🥛🥛🥛
DAY: 7	🥛🥛🥛🥛🥛🥛🥛🥛
DAY: 8	🥛🥛🥛🥛🥛🥛🥛🥛
DAY: 9	🥛🥛🥛🥛🥛🥛🥛🥛
DAY: 10	🥛🥛🥛🥛🥛🥛🥛🥛
DAY: 11	🥛🥛🥛🥛🥛🥛🥛🥛
DAY: 12	🥛🥛🥛🥛🥛🥛🥛🥛
DAY: 13	🥛🥛🥛🥛🥛🥛🥛🥛
DAY: 14	🥛🥛🥛🥛🥛🥛🥛🥛
DAY: 15	🥛🥛🥛🥛🥛🥛🥛🥛

DAY: 16	🥛🥛🥛🥛🥛🥛🥛🥛
DAY: 17	🥛🥛🥛🥛🥛🥛🥛🥛
DAY: 18	🥛🥛🥛🥛🥛🥛🥛🥛
DAY: 19	🥛🥛🥛🥛🥛🥛🥛🥛
DAY: 20	🥛🥛🥛🥛🥛🥛🥛🥛
DAY: 21	🥛🥛🥛🥛🥛🥛🥛🥛
DAY: 22	🥛🥛🥛🥛🥛🥛🥛🥛
DAY: 23	🥛🥛🥛🥛🥛🥛🥛🥛
DAY: 24	🥛🥛🥛🥛🥛🥛🥛🥛
DAY: 25	🥛🥛🥛🥛🥛🥛🥛🥛
DAY: 26	🥛🥛🥛🥛🥛🥛🥛🥛
DAY: 27	🥛🥛🥛🥛🥛🥛🥛🥛
DAY: 28	🥛🥛🥛🥛🥛🥛🥛🥛
DAY: 29	🥛🥛🥛🥛🥛🥛🥛🥛
DAY: 30	🥛🥛🥛🥛🥛🥛🥛🥛

30 DAY
WATER
challenge

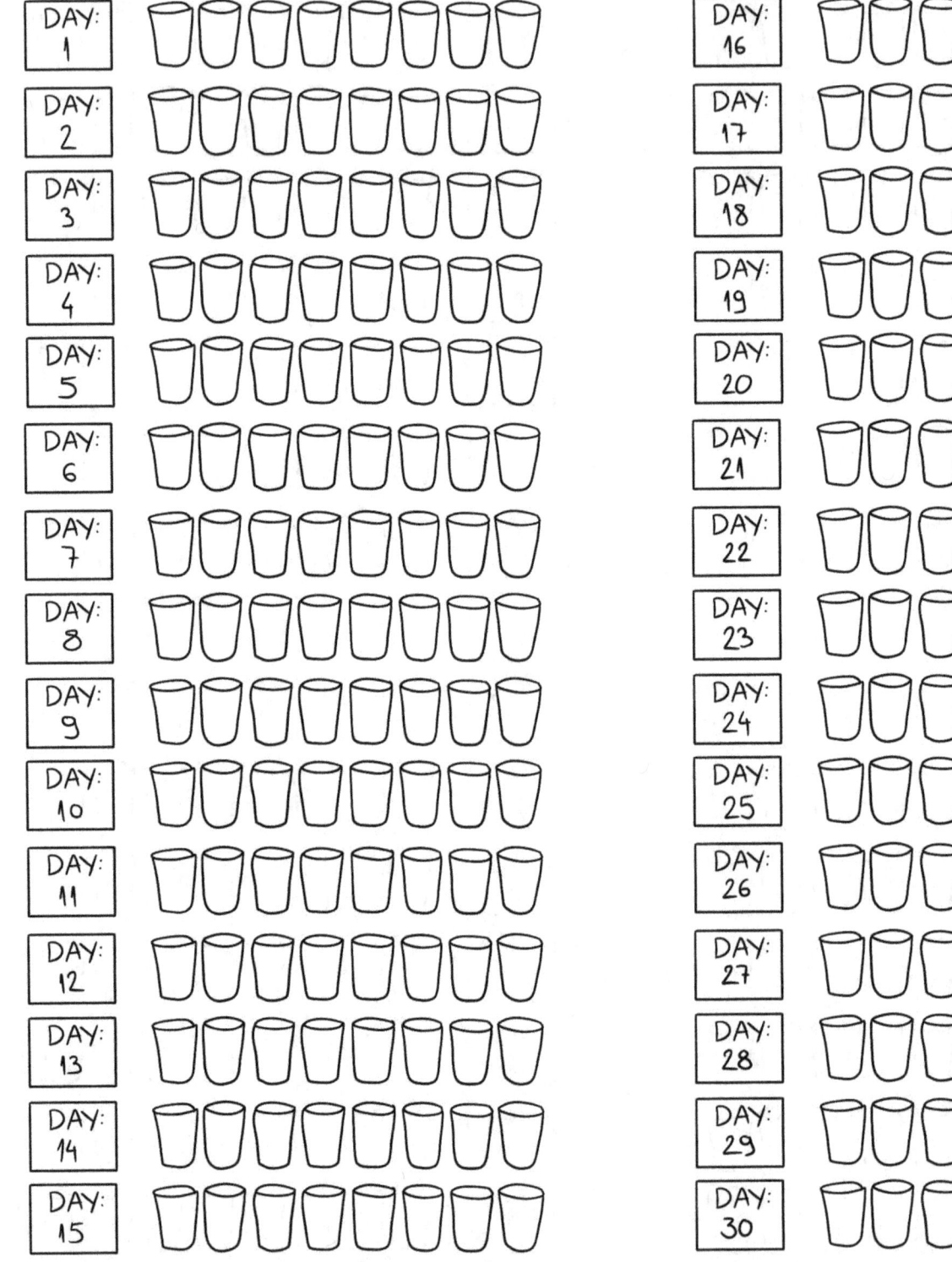

DAY: 1	DAY: 16
DAY: 2	DAY: 17
DAY: 3	DAY: 18
DAY: 4	DAY: 19
DAY: 5	DAY: 20
DAY: 6	DAY: 21
DAY: 7	DAY: 22
DAY: 8	DAY: 23
DAY: 9	DAY: 24
DAY: 10	DAY: 25
DAY: 11	DAY: 26
DAY: 12	DAY: 27
DAY: 13	DAY: 28
DAY: 14	DAY: 29
DAY: 15	DAY: 30

30 DAY
WATER
challenge

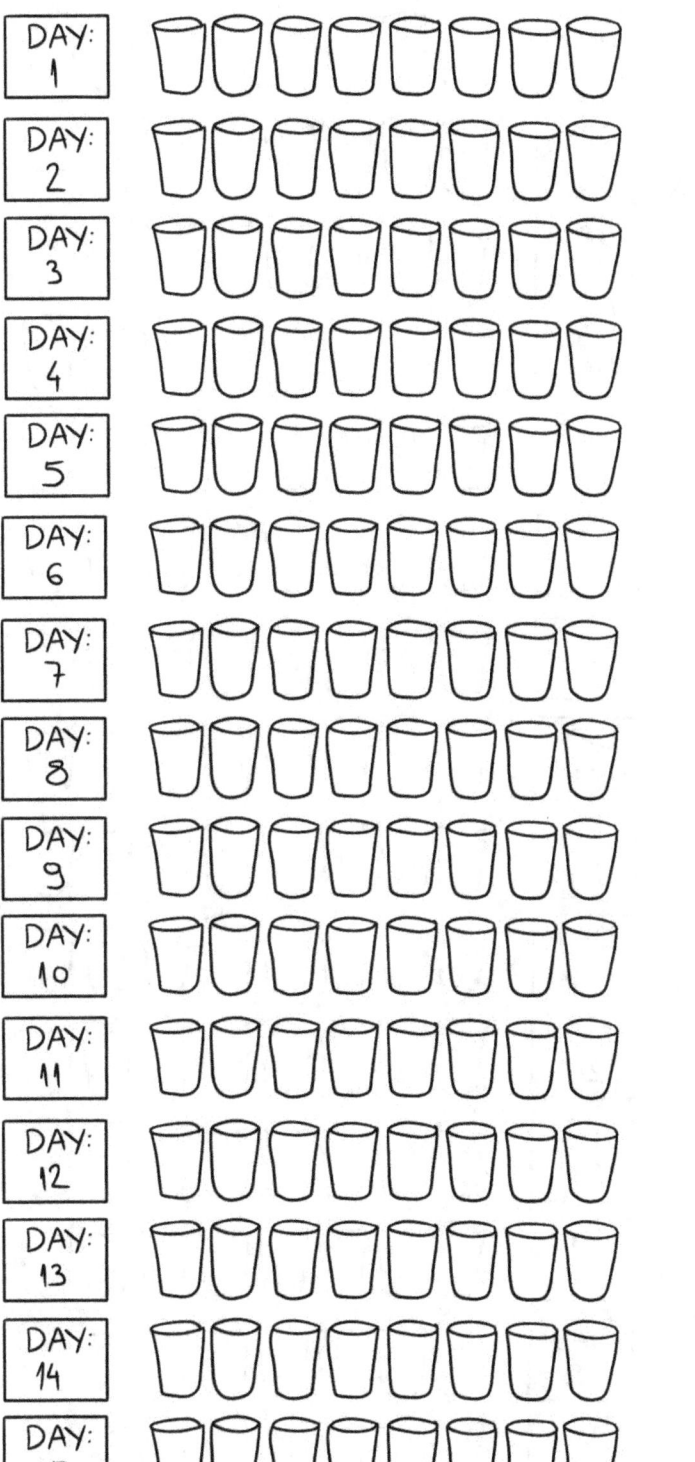

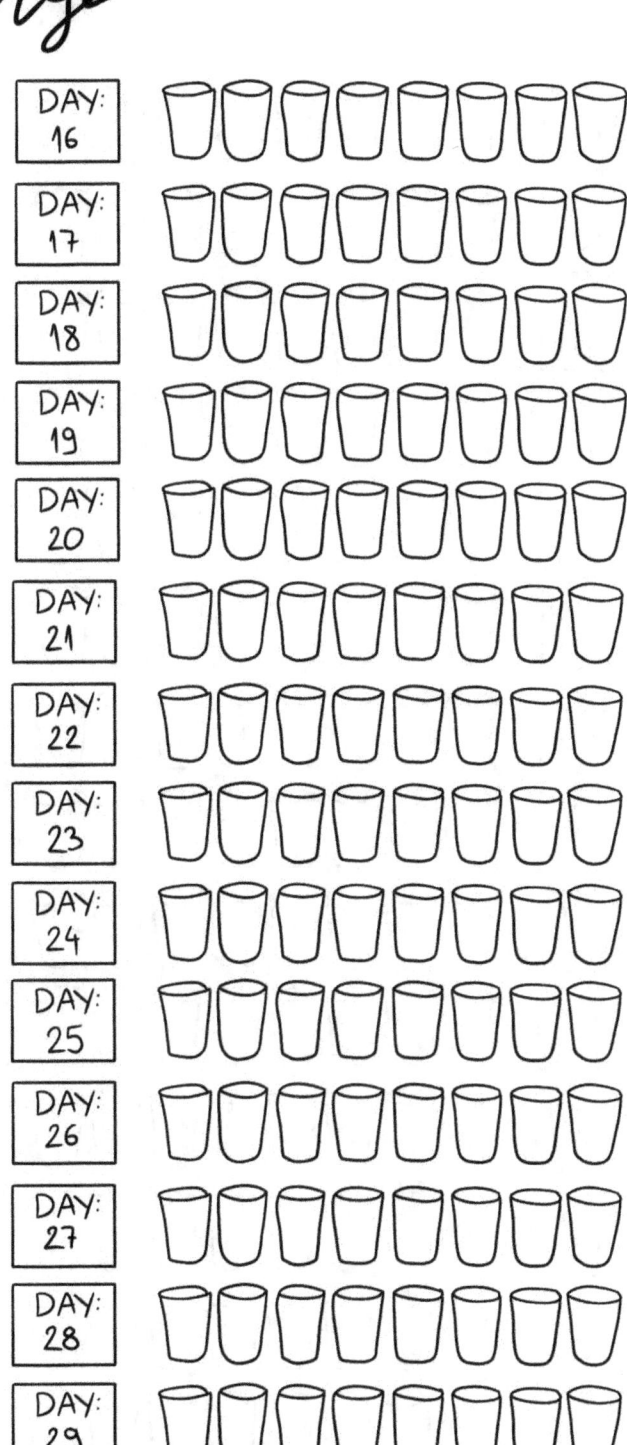

30 DAY
WATER
challenge

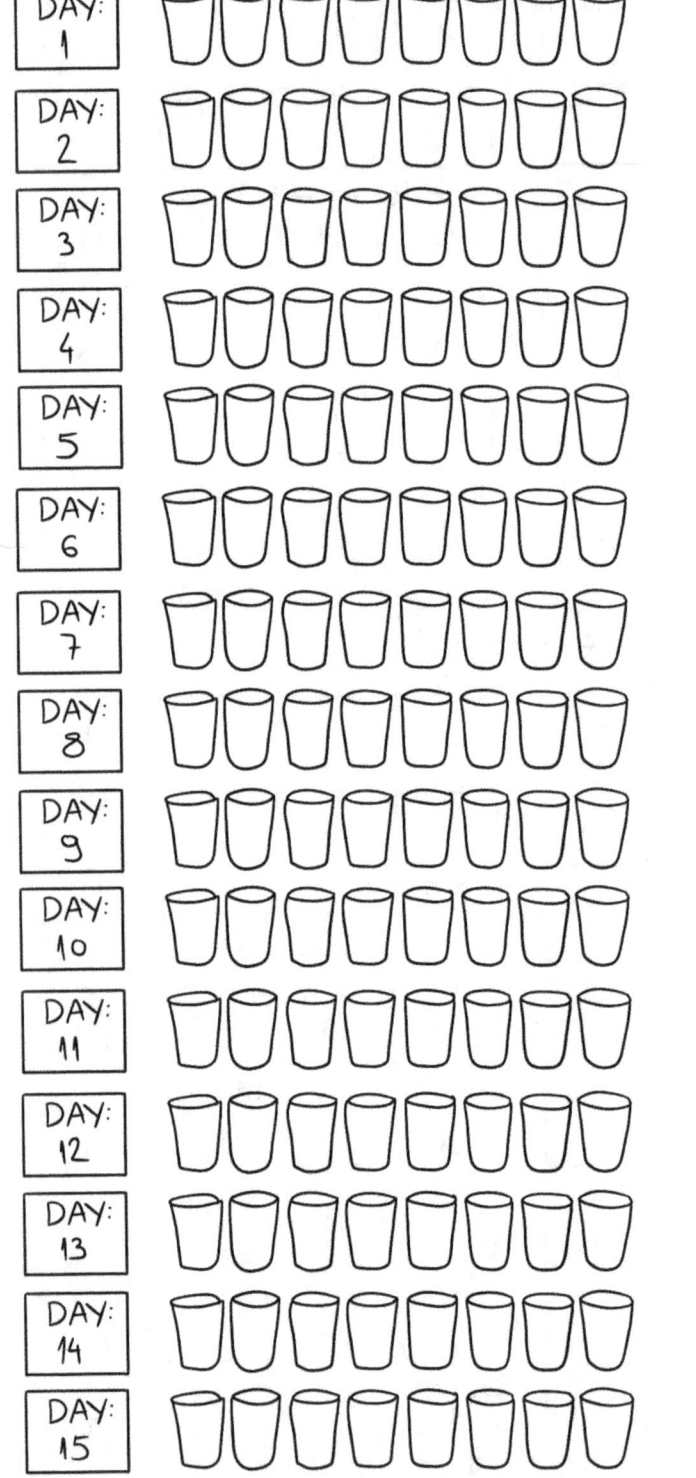

DAY: 1								
DAY: 2								
DAY: 3								
DAY: 4								
DAY: 5								
DAY: 6								
DAY: 7								
DAY: 8								
DAY: 9								
DAY: 10								
DAY: 11								
DAY: 12								
DAY: 13								
DAY: 14								
DAY: 15								

DAY: 16								
DAY: 17								
DAY: 18								
DAY: 19								
DAY: 20								
DAY: 21								
DAY: 22								
DAY: 23								
DAY: 24								
DAY: 25								
DAY: 26								
DAY: 27								
DAY: 28								
DAY: 29								
DAY: 30								

30 DAY
WATER
challenge

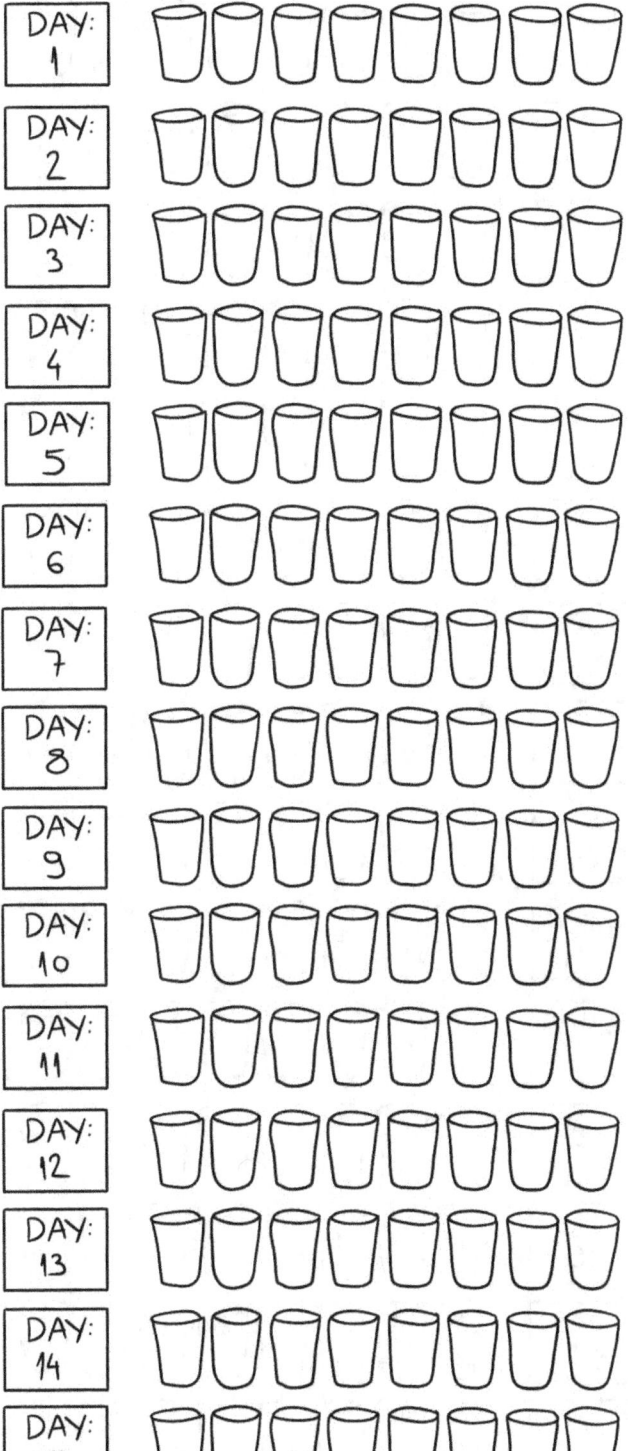

DAY: 1		DAY: 16	
DAY: 2		DAY: 17	
DAY: 3		DAY: 18	
DAY: 4		DAY: 19	
DAY: 5		DAY: 20	
DAY: 6		DAY: 21	
DAY: 7		DAY: 22	
DAY: 8		DAY: 23	
DAY: 9		DAY: 24	
DAY: 10		DAY: 25	
DAY: 11		DAY: 26	
DAY: 12		DAY: 27	
DAY: 13		DAY: 28	
DAY: 14		DAY: 29	
DAY: 15		DAY: 30	

30 DAY
WATER
challenge

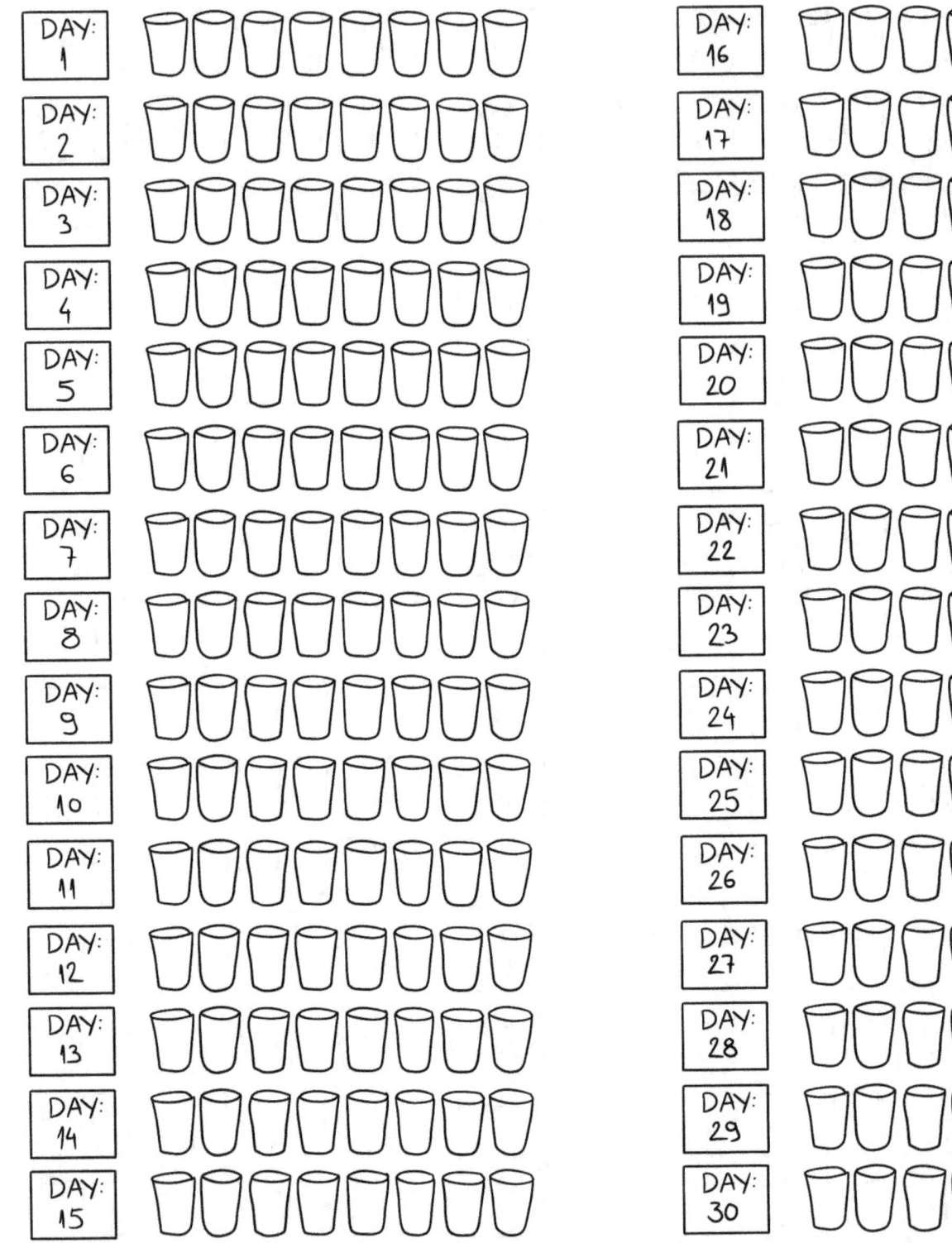

DAY: 1	DAY: 16
DAY: 2	DAY: 17
DAY: 3	DAY: 18
DAY: 4	DAY: 19
DAY: 5	DAY: 20
DAY: 6	DAY: 21
DAY: 7	DAY: 22
DAY: 8	DAY: 23
DAY: 9	DAY: 24
DAY: 10	DAY: 25
DAY: 11	DAY: 26
DAY: 12	DAY: 27
DAY: 13	DAY: 28
DAY: 14	DAY: 29
DAY: 15	DAY: 30

30 DAY
WATER
challenge

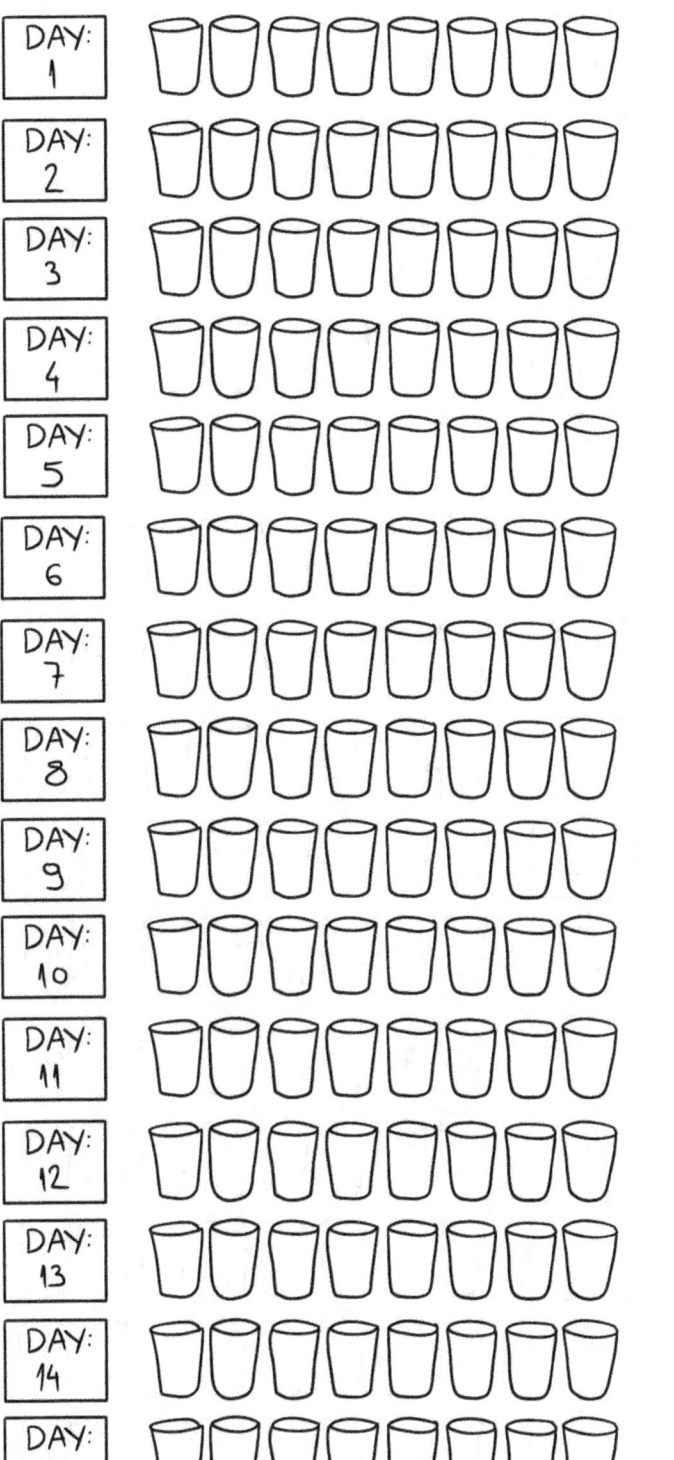

DAY: 1	🥛🥛🥛🥛🥛🥛🥛🥛
DAY: 2	🥛🥛🥛🥛🥛🥛🥛🥛
DAY: 3	🥛🥛🥛🥛🥛🥛🥛🥛
DAY: 4	🥛🥛🥛🥛🥛🥛🥛🥛
DAY: 5	🥛🥛🥛🥛🥛🥛🥛🥛
DAY: 6	🥛🥛🥛🥛🥛🥛🥛🥛
DAY: 7	🥛🥛🥛🥛🥛🥛🥛🥛
DAY: 8	🥛🥛🥛🥛🥛🥛🥛🥛
DAY: 9	🥛🥛🥛🥛🥛🥛🥛🥛
DAY: 10	🥛🥛🥛🥛🥛🥛🥛🥛
DAY: 11	🥛🥛🥛🥛🥛🥛🥛🥛
DAY: 12	🥛🥛🥛🥛🥛🥛🥛🥛
DAY: 13	🥛🥛🥛🥛🥛🥛🥛🥛
DAY: 14	🥛🥛🥛🥛🥛🥛🥛🥛
DAY: 15	🥛🥛🥛🥛🥛🥛🥛🥛
DAY: 16	🥛🥛🥛🥛🥛🥛🥛🥛
DAY: 17	🥛🥛🥛🥛🥛🥛🥛🥛
DAY: 18	🥛🥛🥛🥛🥛🥛🥛🥛
DAY: 19	🥛🥛🥛🥛🥛🥛🥛🥛
DAY: 20	🥛🥛🥛🥛🥛🥛🥛🥛
DAY: 21	🥛🥛🥛🥛🥛🥛🥛🥛
DAY: 22	🥛🥛🥛🥛🥛🥛🥛🥛
DAY: 23	🥛🥛🥛🥛🥛🥛🥛🥛
DAY: 24	🥛🥛🥛🥛🥛🥛🥛🥛
DAY: 25	🥛🥛🥛🥛🥛🥛🥛🥛
DAY: 26	🥛🥛🥛🥛🥛🥛🥛🥛
DAY: 27	🥛🥛🥛🥛🥛🥛🥛🥛
DAY: 28	🥛🥛🥛🥛🥛🥛🥛🥛
DAY: 29	🥛🥛🥛🥛🥛🥛🥛🥛
DAY: 30	🥛🥛🥛🥛🥛🥛🥛🥛

30 DAY
WATER
challenge

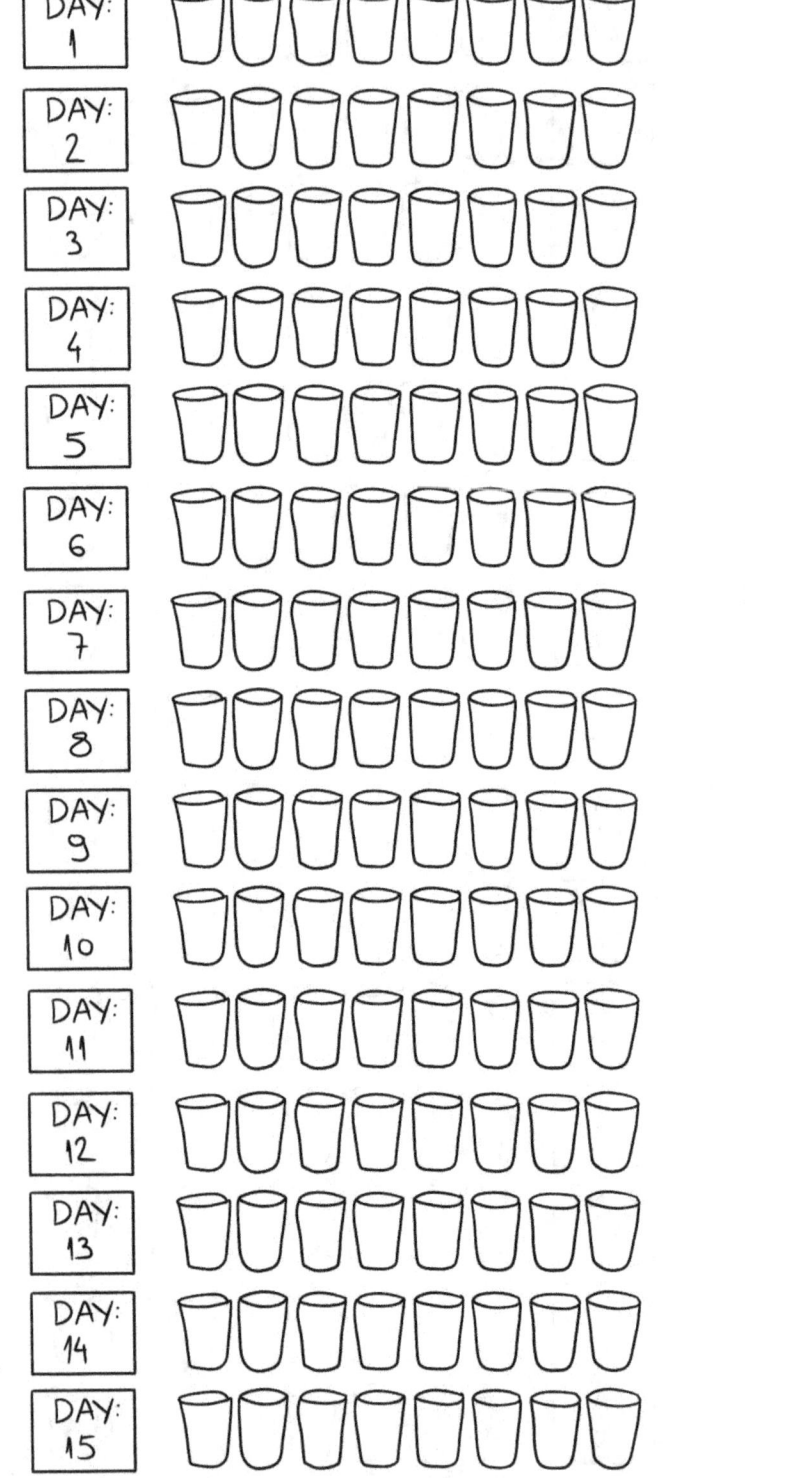

DAY: 1								
DAY: 2								
DAY: 3								
DAY: 4								
DAY: 5								
DAY: 6								
DAY: 7								
DAY: 8								
DAY: 9								
DAY: 10								
DAY: 11								
DAY: 12								
DAY: 13								
DAY: 14								
DAY: 15								

DAY: 16								
DAY: 17								
DAY: 18								
DAY: 19								
DAY: 20								
DAY: 21								
DAY: 22								
DAY: 23								
DAY: 24								
DAY: 25								
DAY: 26								
DAY: 27								
DAY: 28								
DAY: 29								
DAY: 30								

30 DAY
WATER
challenge

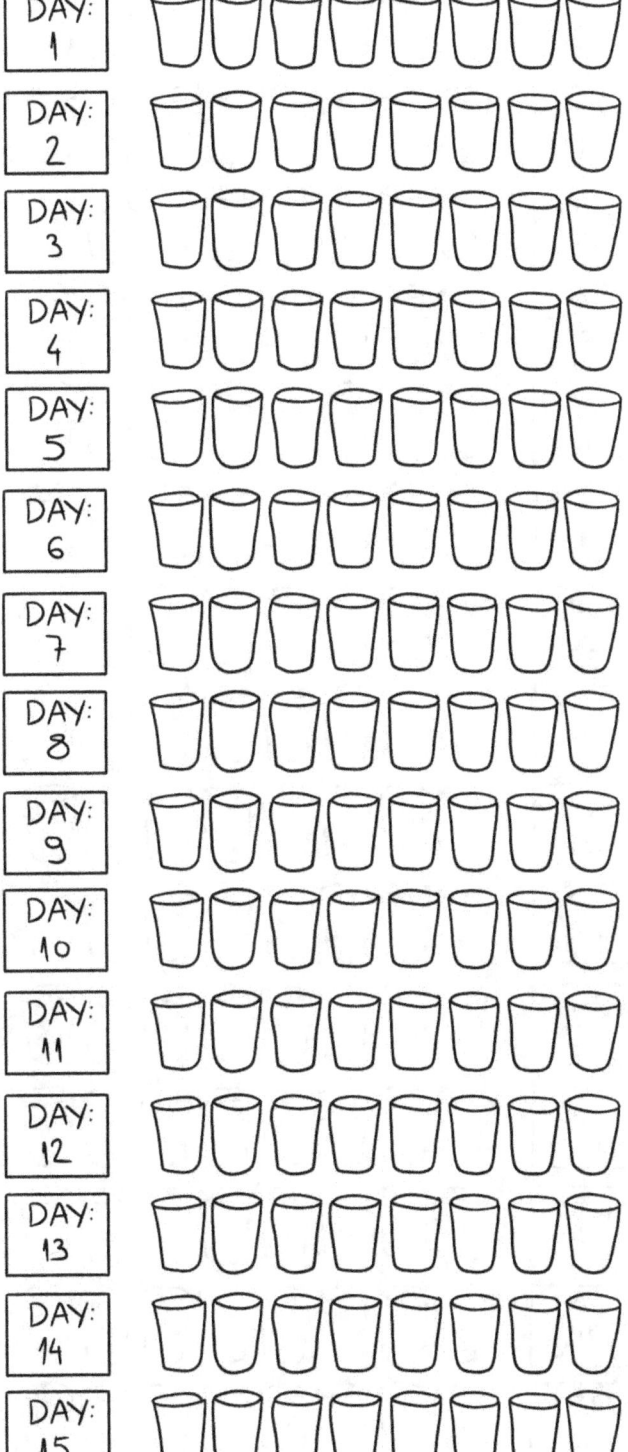

DAY: 1							
DAY: 2							
DAY: 3							
DAY: 4							
DAY: 5							
DAY: 6							
DAY: 7							
DAY: 8							
DAY: 9							
DAY: 10							
DAY: 11							
DAY: 12							
DAY: 13							
DAY: 14							
DAY: 15							

DAY: 16							
DAY: 17							
DAY: 18							
DAY: 19							
DAY: 20							
DAY: 21							
DAY: 22							
DAY: 23							
DAY: 24							
DAY: 25							
DAY: 26							
DAY: 27							
DAY: 28							
DAY: 29							
DAY: 30							

30 DAY WATER
challenge

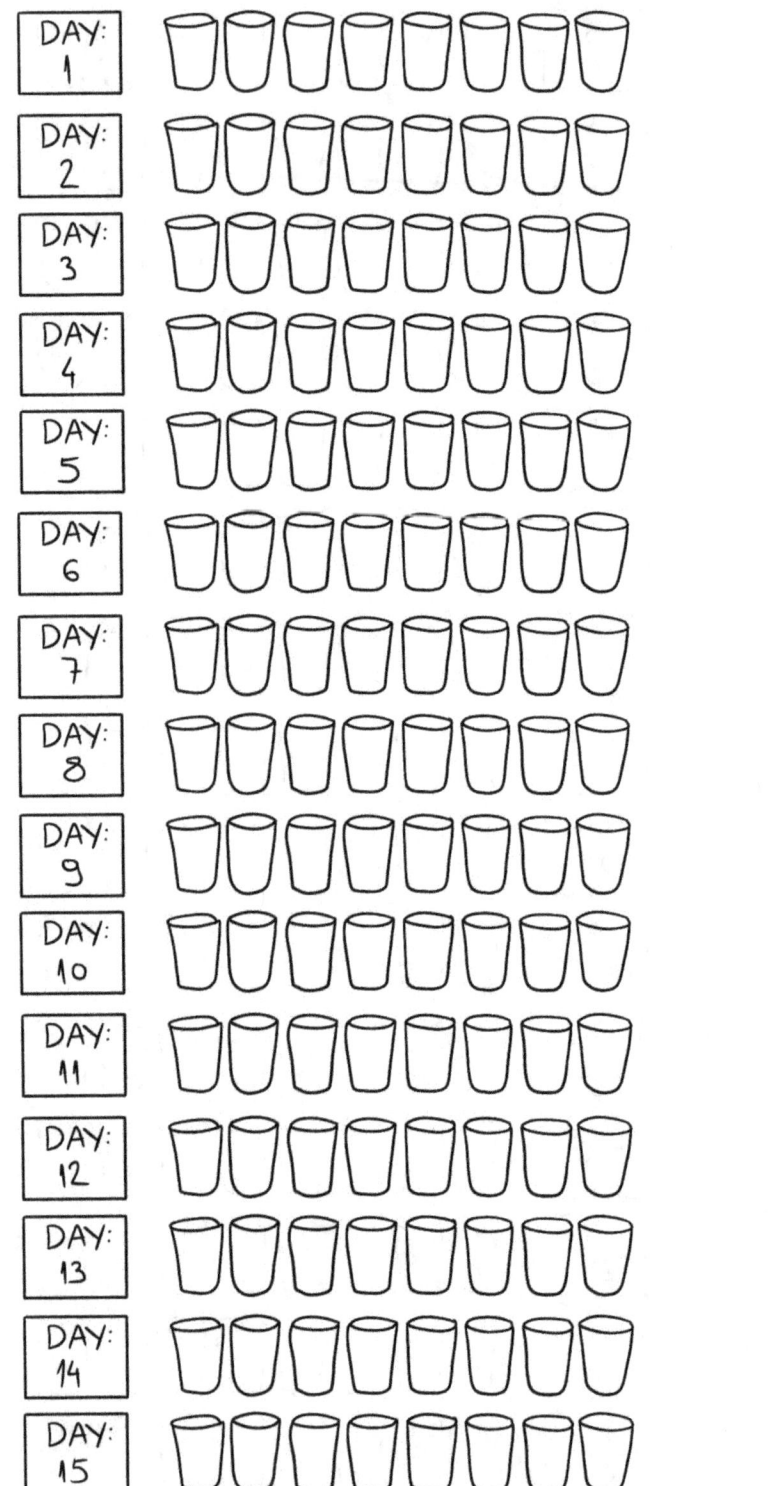

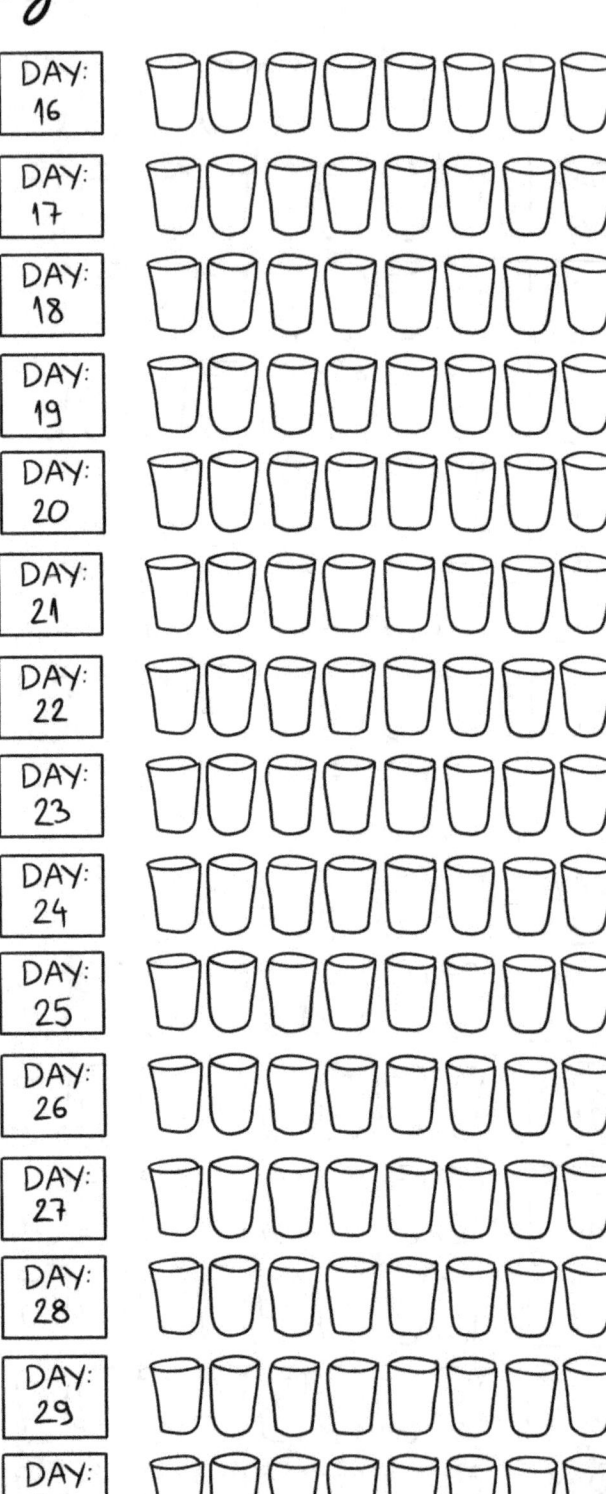

30 DAY
WATER
challenge

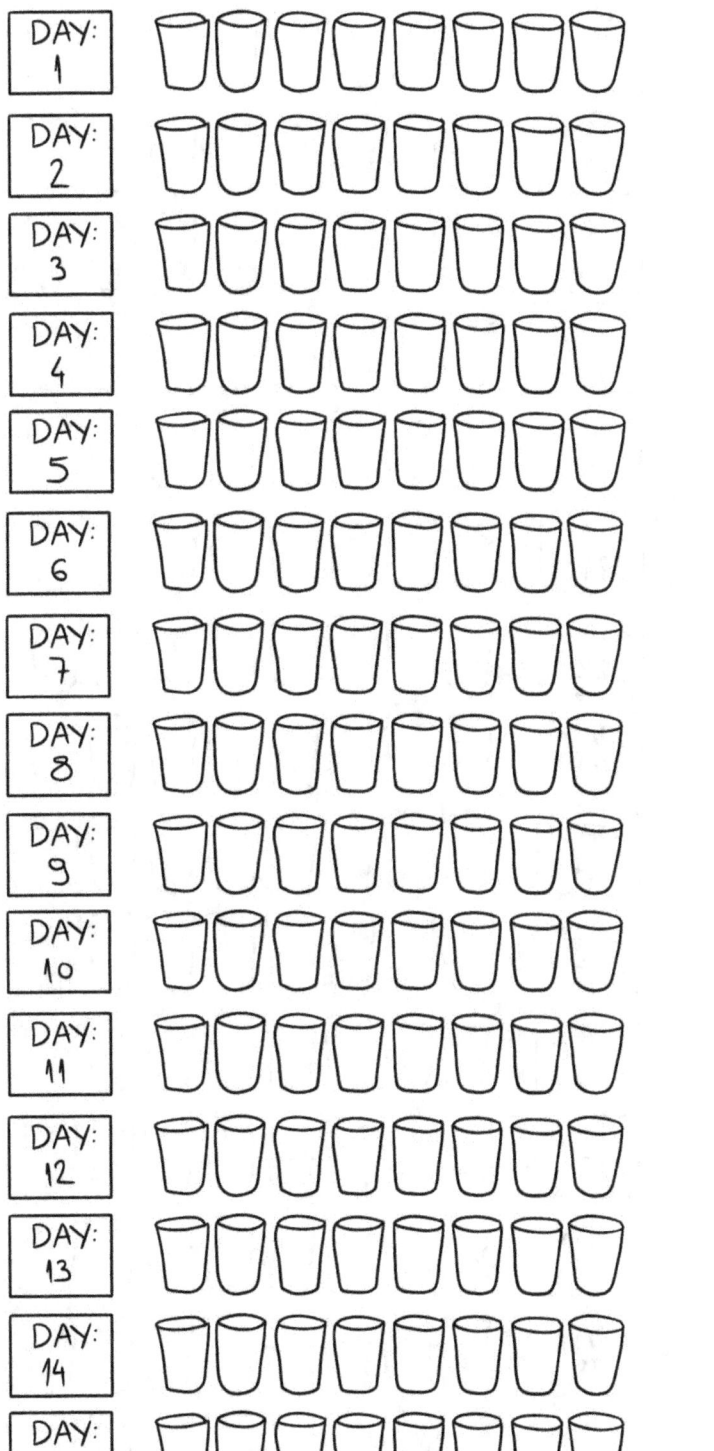
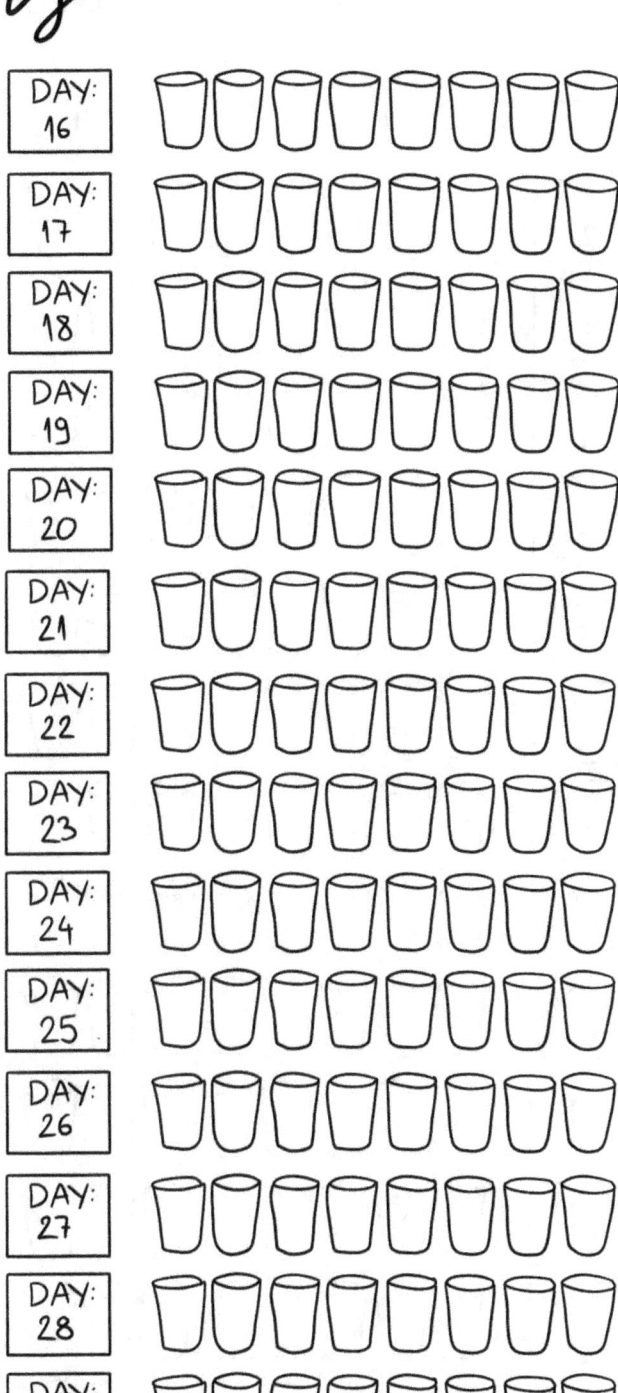

DAY: 1		DAY: 16
DAY: 2		DAY: 17
DAY: 3		DAY: 18
DAY: 4		DAY: 19
DAY: 5		DAY: 20
DAY: 6		DAY: 21
DAY: 7		DAY: 22
DAY: 8		DAY: 23
DAY: 9		DAY: 24
DAY: 10		DAY: 25
DAY: 11		DAY: 26
DAY: 12		DAY: 27
DAY: 13		DAY: 28
DAY: 14		DAY: 29
DAY: 15		DAY: 30

30 DAY WATER challenge

DAY: 1	⊔⊔⊔⊔⊔⊔⊔⊔	DAY: 16	⊔⊔⊔⊔⊔⊔⊔⊔
DAY: 2	⊔⊔⊔⊔⊔⊔⊔⊔	DAY: 17	⊔⊔⊔⊔⊔⊔⊔⊔
DAY: 3	⊔⊔⊔⊔⊔⊔⊔⊔	DAY: 18	⊔⊔⊔⊔⊔⊔⊔⊔
DAY: 4	⊔⊔⊔⊔⊔⊔⊔⊔	DAY: 19	⊔⊔⊔⊔⊔⊔⊔⊔
DAY: 5	⊔⊔⊔⊔⊔⊔⊔⊔	DAY: 20	⊔⊔⊔⊔⊔⊔⊔⊔
DAY: 6	⊔⊔⊔⊔⊔⊔⊔⊔	DAY: 21	⊔⊔⊔⊔⊔⊔⊔⊔
DAY: 7	⊔⊔⊔⊔⊔⊔⊔⊔	DAY: 22	⊔⊔⊔⊔⊔⊔⊔⊔
DAY: 8	⊔⊔⊔⊔⊔⊔⊔⊔	DAY: 23	⊔⊔⊔⊔⊔⊔⊔⊔
DAY: 9	⊔⊔⊔⊔⊔⊔⊔⊔	DAY: 24	⊔⊔⊔⊔⊔⊔⊔⊔
DAY: 10	⊔⊔⊔⊔⊔⊔⊔⊔	DAY: 25	⊔⊔⊔⊔⊔⊔⊔⊔
DAY: 11	⊔⊔⊔⊔⊔⊔⊔⊔	DAY: 26	⊔⊔⊔⊔⊔⊔⊔⊔
DAY: 12	⊔⊔⊔⊔⊔⊔⊔⊔	DAY: 27	⊔⊔⊔⊔⊔⊔⊔⊔
DAY: 13	⊔⊔⊔⊔⊔⊔⊔⊔	DAY: 28	⊔⊔⊔⊔⊔⊔⊔⊔
DAY: 14	⊔⊔⊔⊔⊔⊔⊔⊔	DAY: 29	⊔⊔⊔⊔⊔⊔⊔⊔
DAY: 15	⊔⊔⊔⊔⊔⊔⊔⊔	DAY: 30	⊔⊔⊔⊔⊔⊔⊔⊔

30 DAY
WATER
challenge

DAY: 1								
DAY: 2								
DAY: 3								
DAY: 4								
DAY: 5								
DAY: 6								
DAY: 7								
DAY: 8								
DAY: 9								
DAY: 10								
DAY: 11								
DAY: 12								
DAY: 13								
DAY: 14								
DAY: 15								

DAY: 16								
DAY: 17								
DAY: 18								
DAY: 19								
DAY: 20								
DAY: 21								
DAY: 22								
DAY: 23								
DAY: 24								
DAY: 25								
DAY: 26								
DAY: 27								
DAY: 28								
DAY: 29								
DAY: 30								

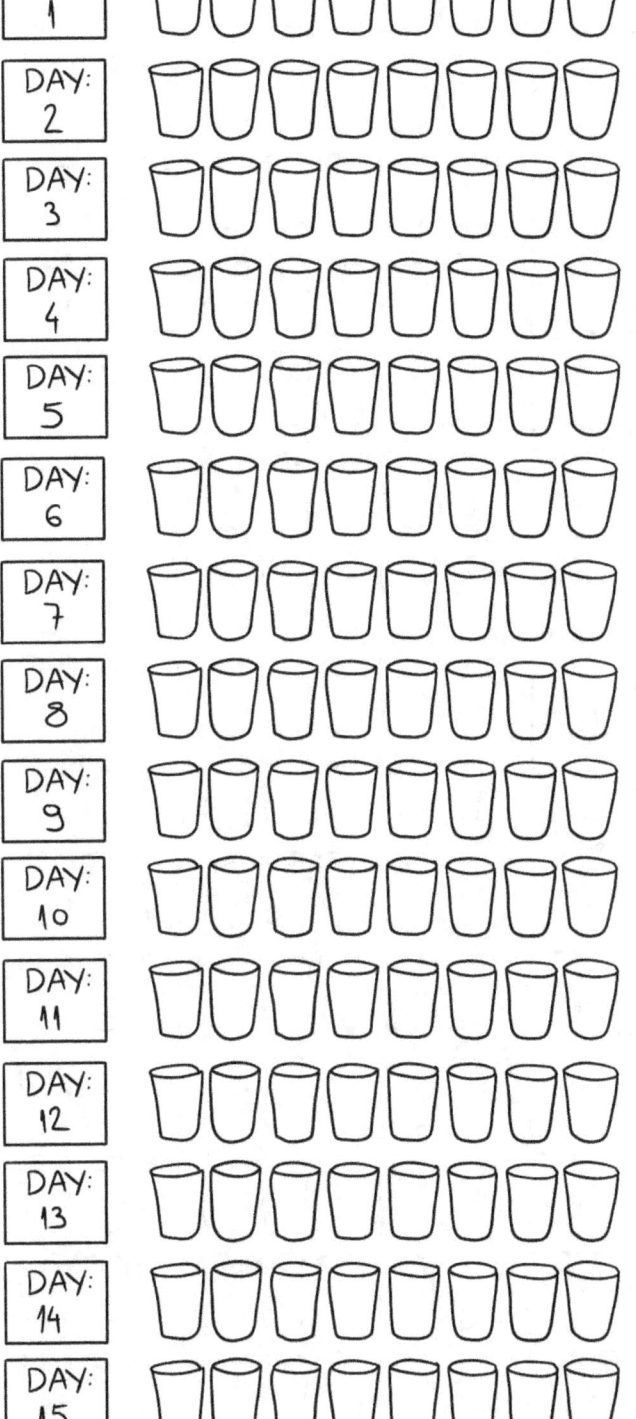

30 DAY
WATER
challenge

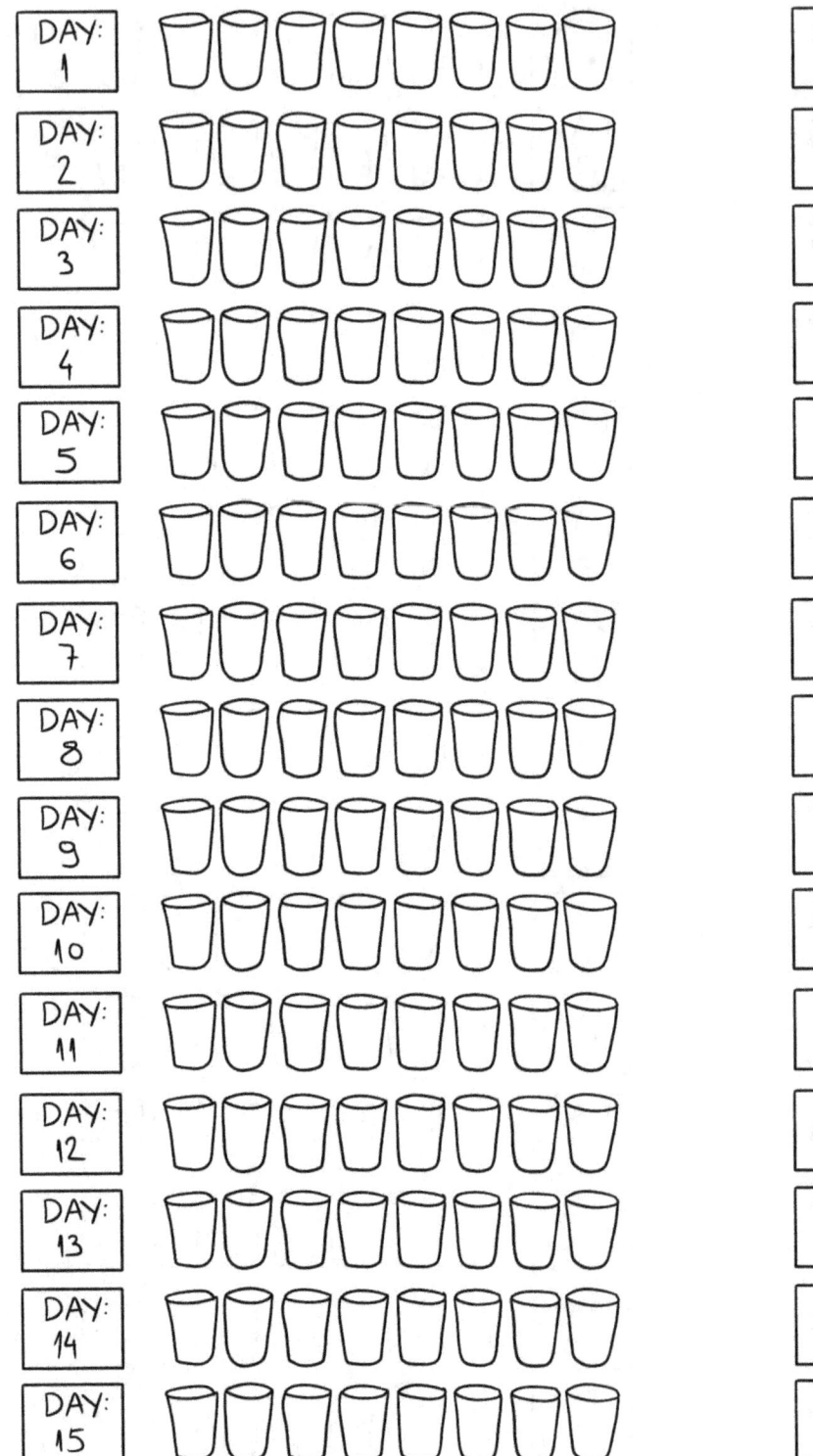

DAY: 1							
DAY: 2							
DAY: 3							
DAY: 4							
DAY: 5							
DAY: 6							
DAY: 7							
DAY: 8							
DAY: 9							
DAY: 10							
DAY: 11							
DAY: 12							
DAY: 13							
DAY: 14							
DAY: 15							

DAY: 16							
DAY: 17							
DAY: 18							
DAY: 19							
DAY: 20							
DAY: 21							
DAY: 22							
DAY: 23							
DAY: 24							
DAY: 25							
DAY: 26							
DAY: 27							
DAY: 28							
DAY: 29							
DAY: 30							

30 DAY
WATER
challenge

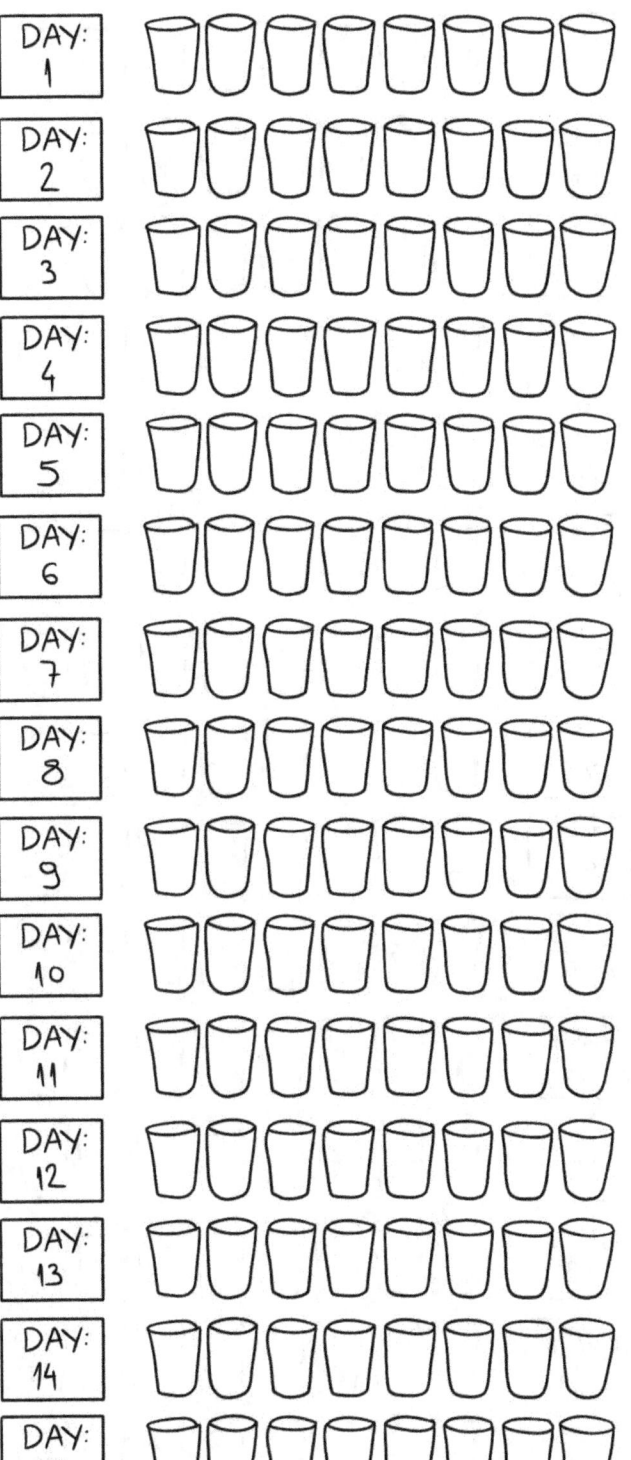

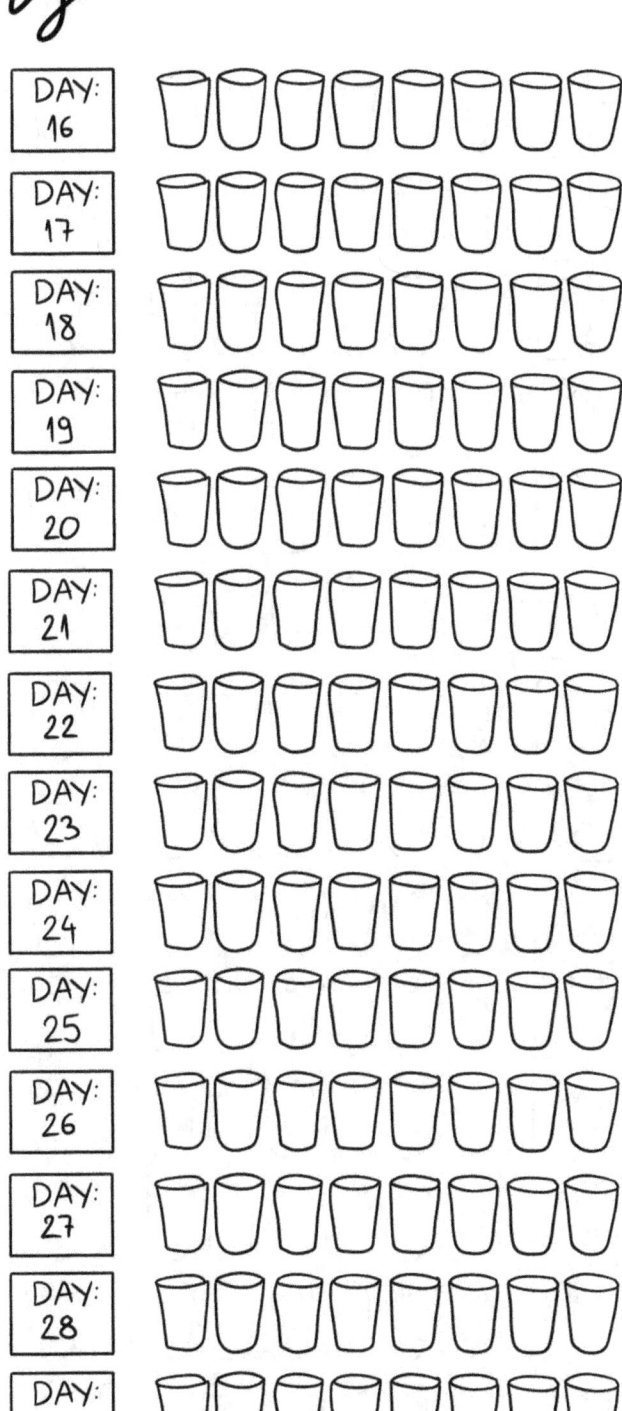

30 DAY WATER challenge

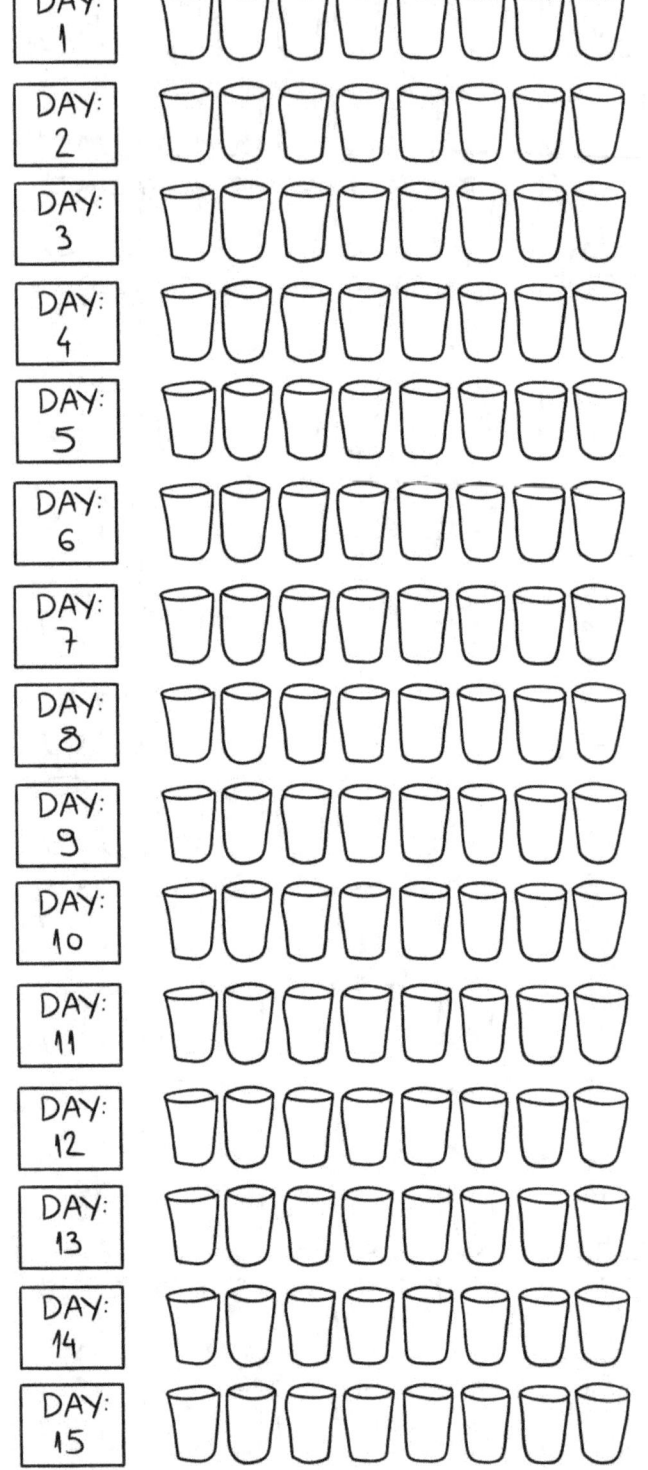

DAY: 1		DAY: 16	
DAY: 2		DAY: 17	
DAY: 3		DAY: 18	
DAY: 4		DAY: 19	
DAY: 5		DAY: 20	
DAY: 6		DAY: 21	
DAY: 7		DAY: 22	
DAY: 8		DAY: 23	
DAY: 9		DAY: 24	
DAY: 10		DAY: 25	
DAY: 11		DAY: 26	
DAY: 12		DAY: 27	
DAY: 13		DAY: 28	
DAY: 14		DAY: 29	
DAY: 15		DAY: 30	

30 DAY
WATER
challenge

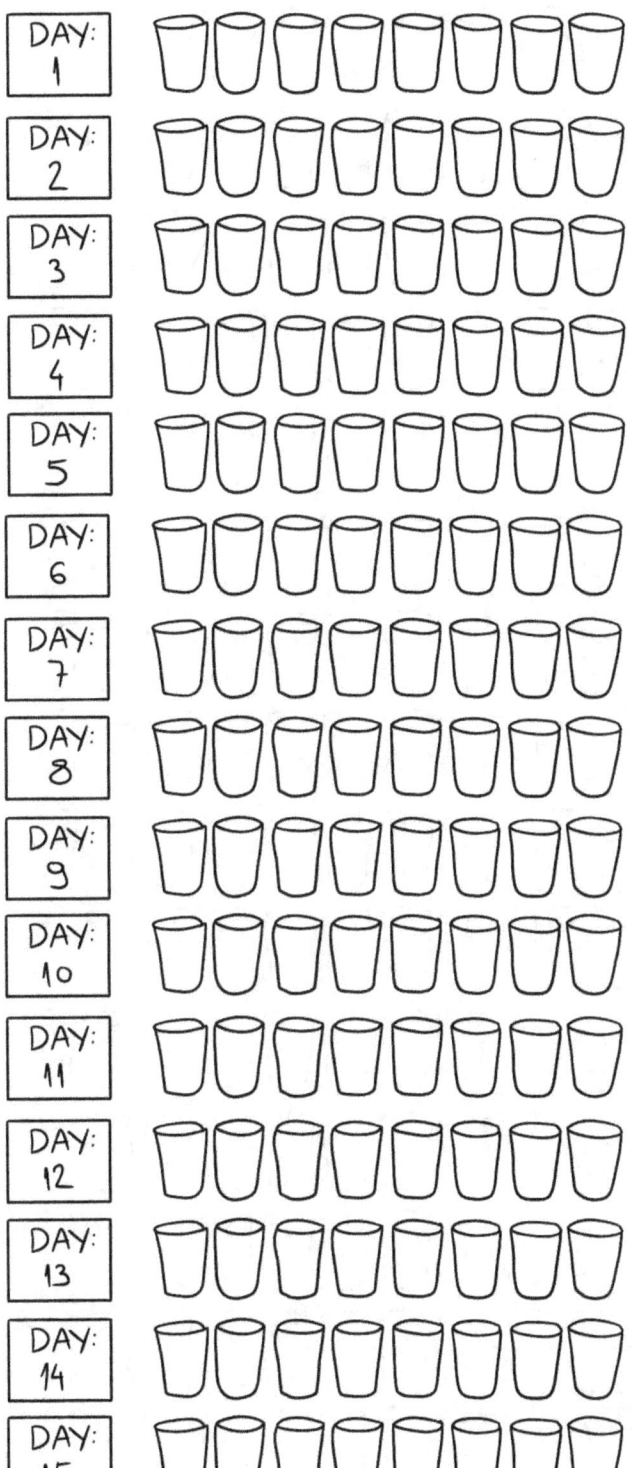
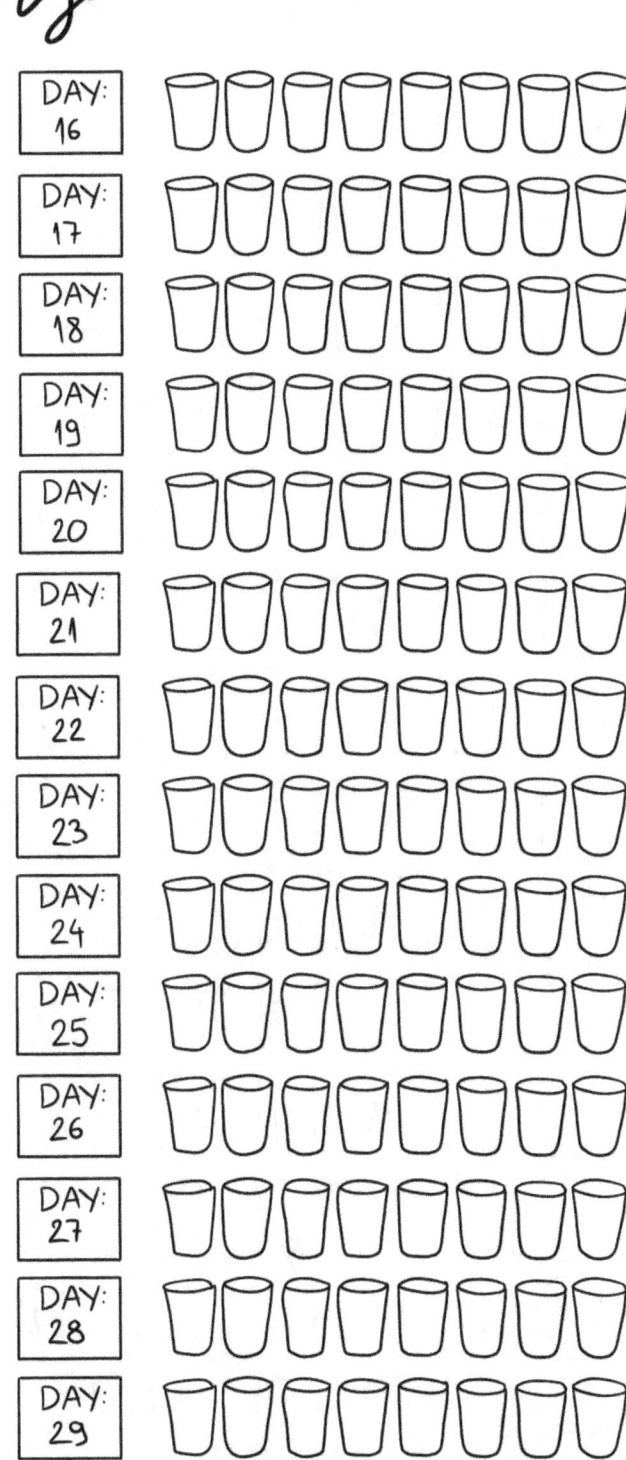

DAY: 1

DAY: 2

DAY: 3

DAY: 4

DAY: 5

DAY: 6

DAY: 7

DAY: 8

DAY: 9

DAY: 10

DAY: 11

DAY: 12

DAY: 13

DAY: 14

DAY: 15

DAY: 16

DAY: 17

DAY: 18

DAY: 19

DAY: 20

DAY: 21

DAY: 22

DAY: 23

DAY: 24

DAY: 25

DAY: 26

DAY: 27

DAY: 28

DAY: 29

DAY: 30

30 DAY
WATER
challenge

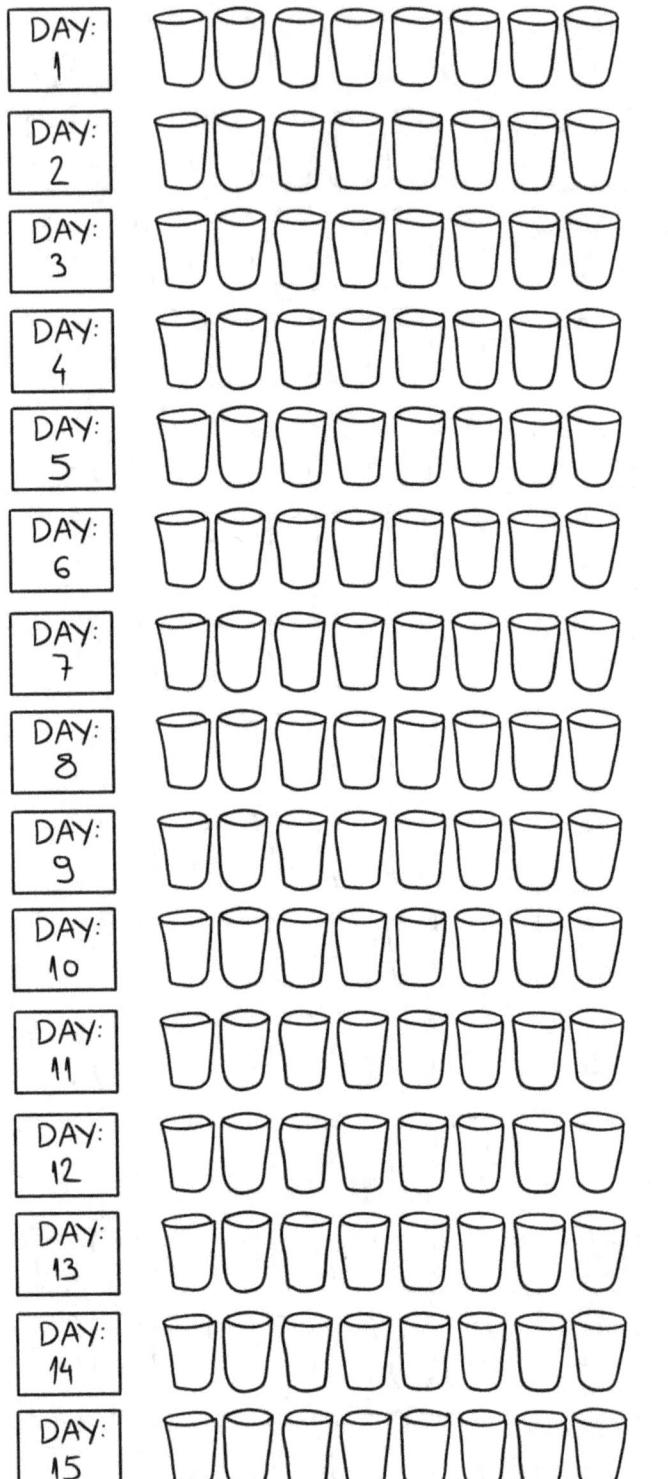

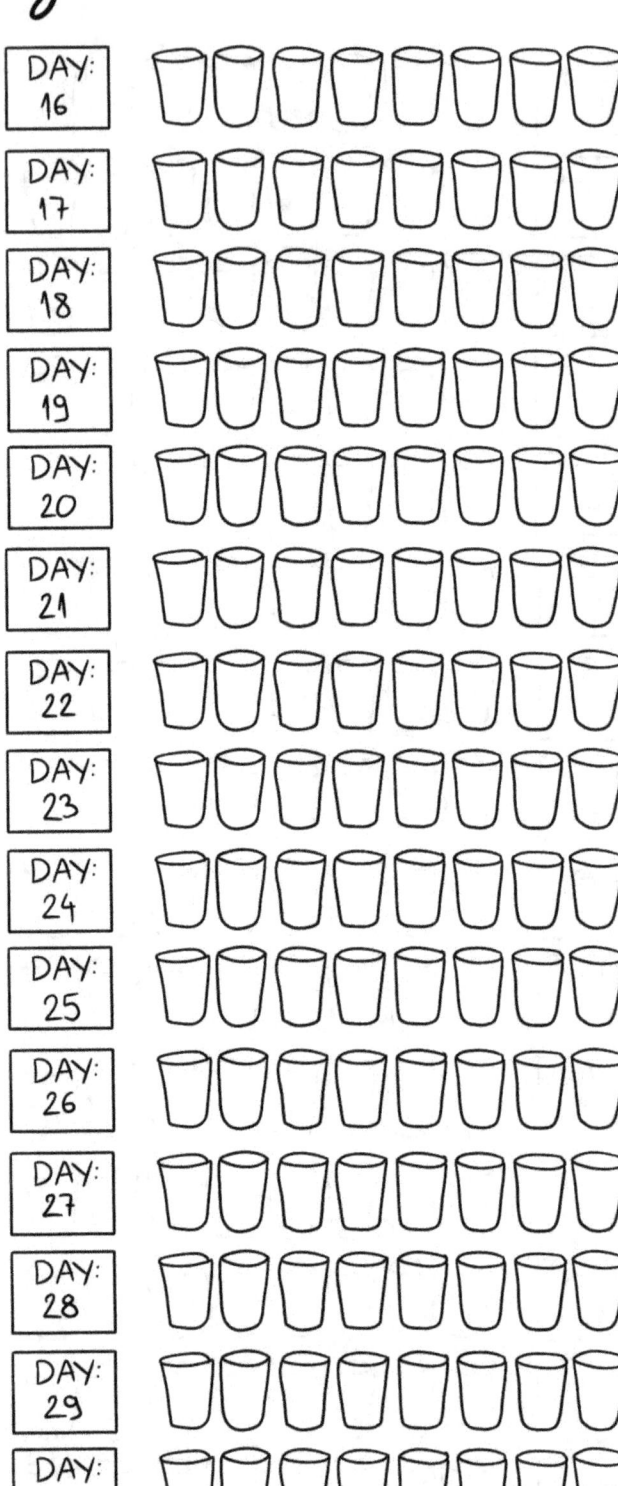

30 DAY
WATER
challenge

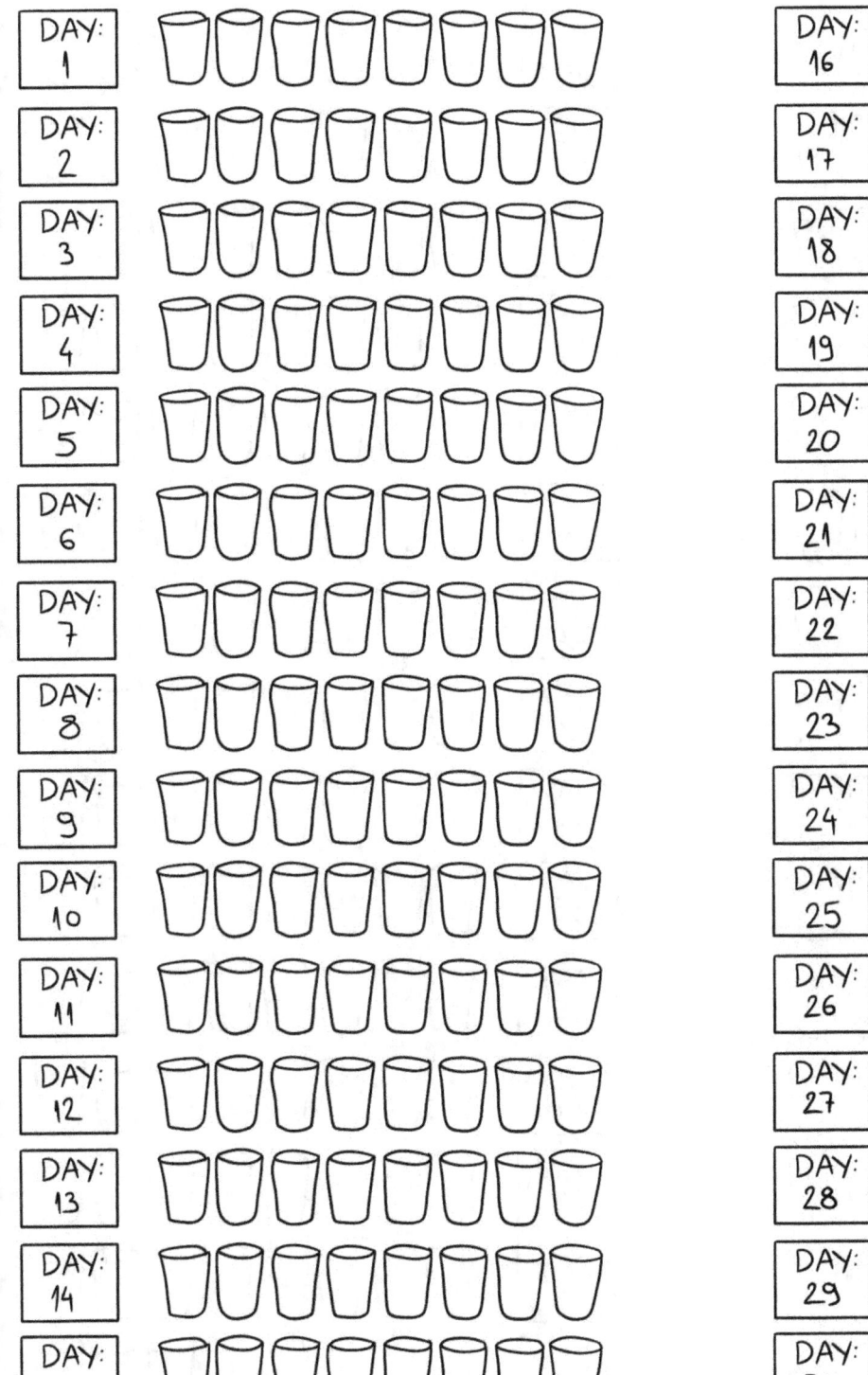

DAY: 1		DAY: 16	
DAY: 2		DAY: 17	
DAY: 3		DAY: 18	
DAY: 4		DAY: 19	
DAY: 5		DAY: 20	
DAY: 6		DAY: 21	
DAY: 7		DAY: 22	
DAY: 8		DAY: 23	
DAY: 9		DAY: 24	
DAY: 10		DAY: 25	
DAY: 11		DAY: 26	
DAY: 12		DAY: 27	
DAY: 13		DAY: 28	
DAY: 14		DAY: 29	
DAY: 15		DAY: 30	

30 DAY
WATER
challenge

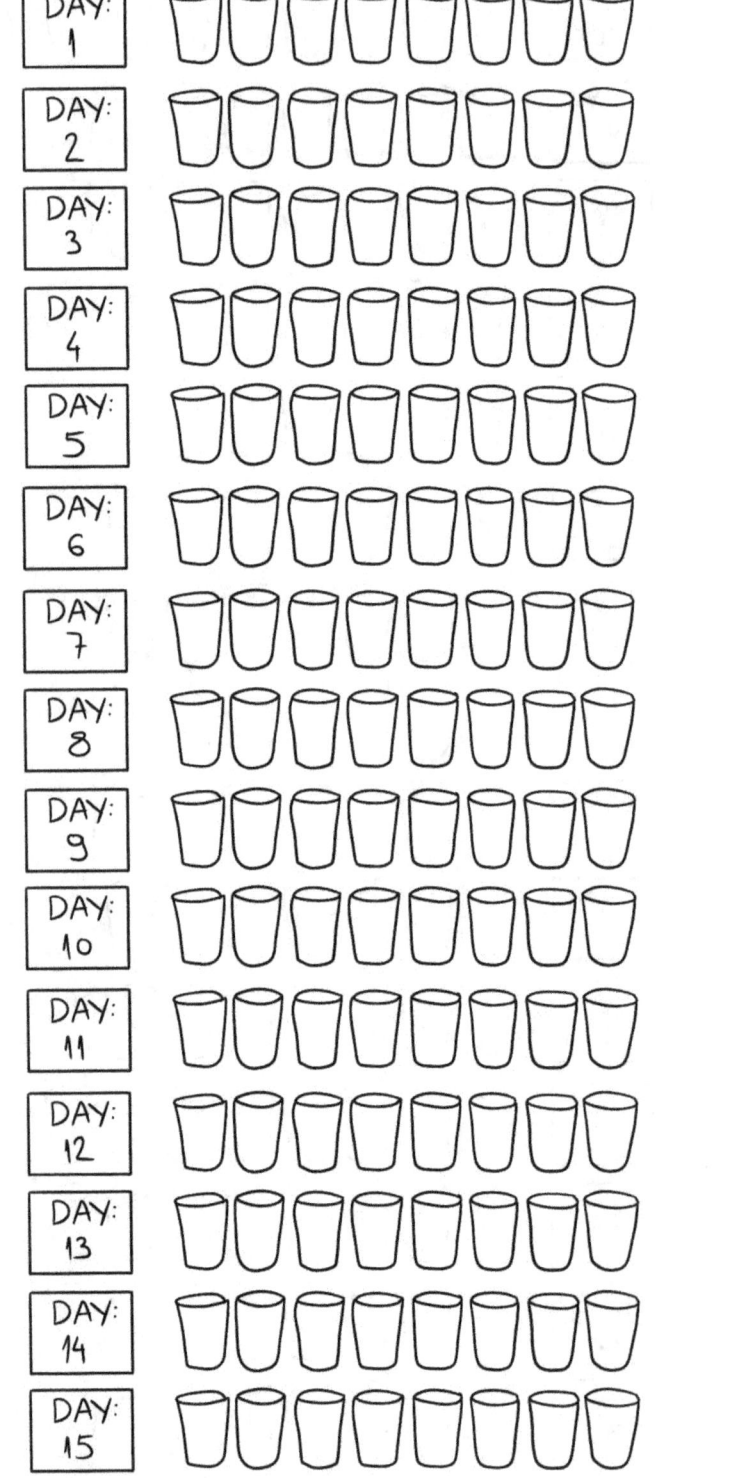

DAY: 1	DAY: 16
DAY: 2	DAY: 17
DAY: 3	DAY: 18
DAY: 4	DAY: 19
DAY: 5	DAY: 20
DAY: 6	DAY: 21
DAY: 7	DAY: 22
DAY: 8	DAY: 23
DAY: 9	DAY: 24
DAY: 10	DAY: 25
DAY: 11	DAY: 26
DAY: 12	DAY: 27
DAY: 13	DAY: 28
DAY: 14	DAY: 29
DAY: 15	DAY: 30

30 DAY
WATER
challenge

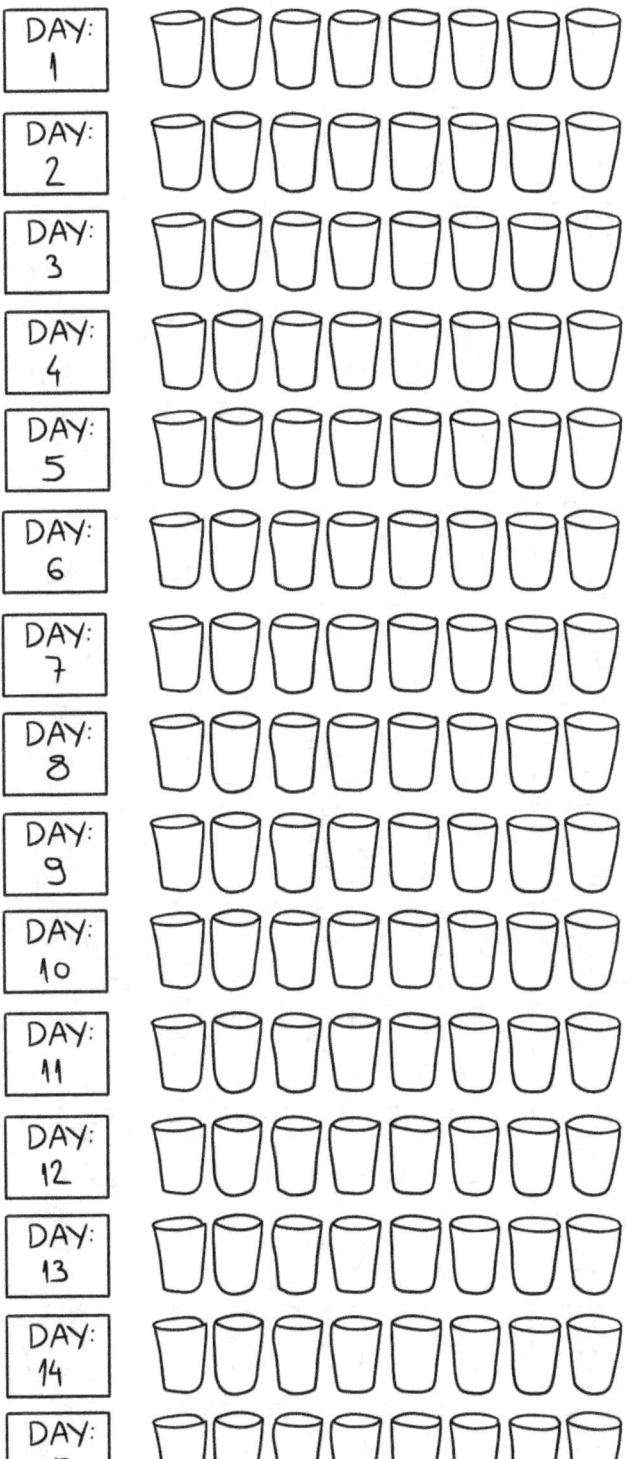

DAY: 1							
DAY: 2							
DAY: 3							
DAY: 4							
DAY: 5							
DAY: 6							
DAY: 7							
DAY: 8							
DAY: 9							
DAY: 10							
DAY: 11							
DAY: 12							
DAY: 13							
DAY: 14							
DAY: 15							

DAY: 16							
DAY: 17							
DAY: 18							
DAY: 19							
DAY: 20							
DAY: 21							
DAY: 22							
DAY: 23							
DAY: 24							
DAY: 25							
DAY: 26							
DAY: 27							
DAY: 28							
DAY: 29							
DAY: 30							

30 DAY
WATER
challenge

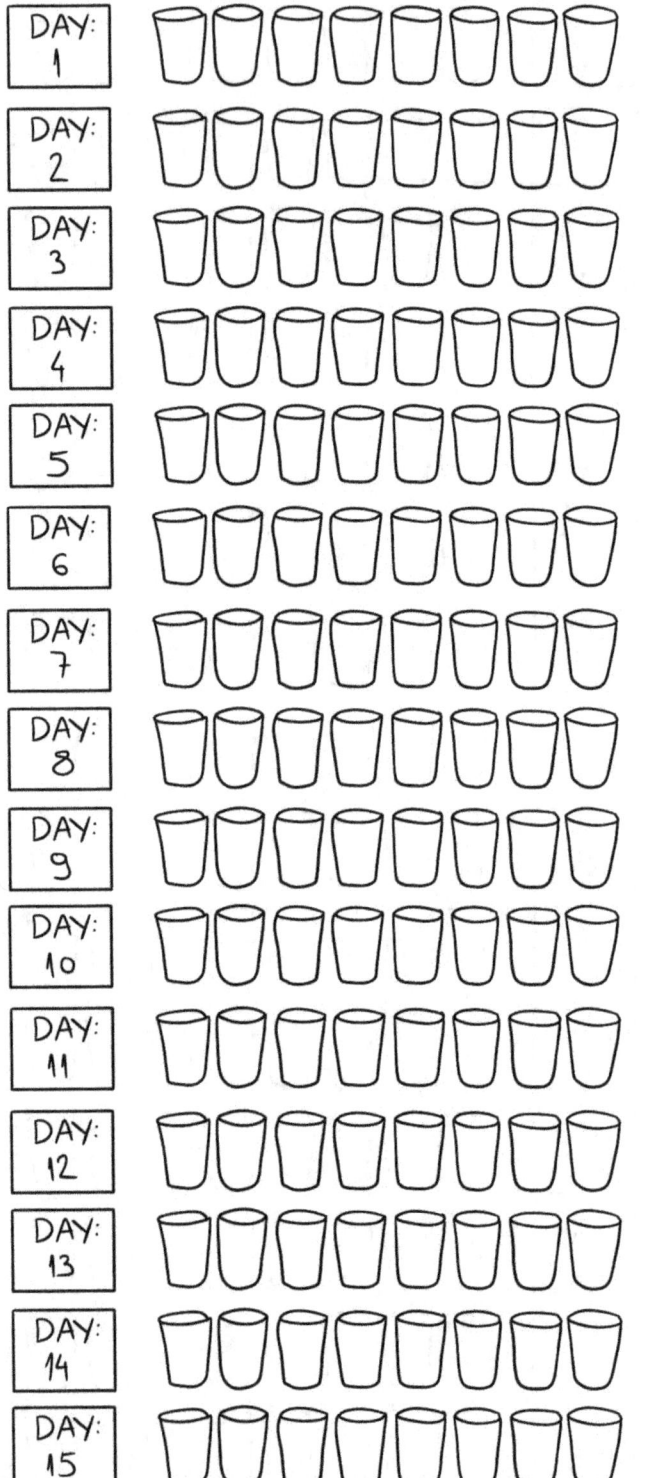

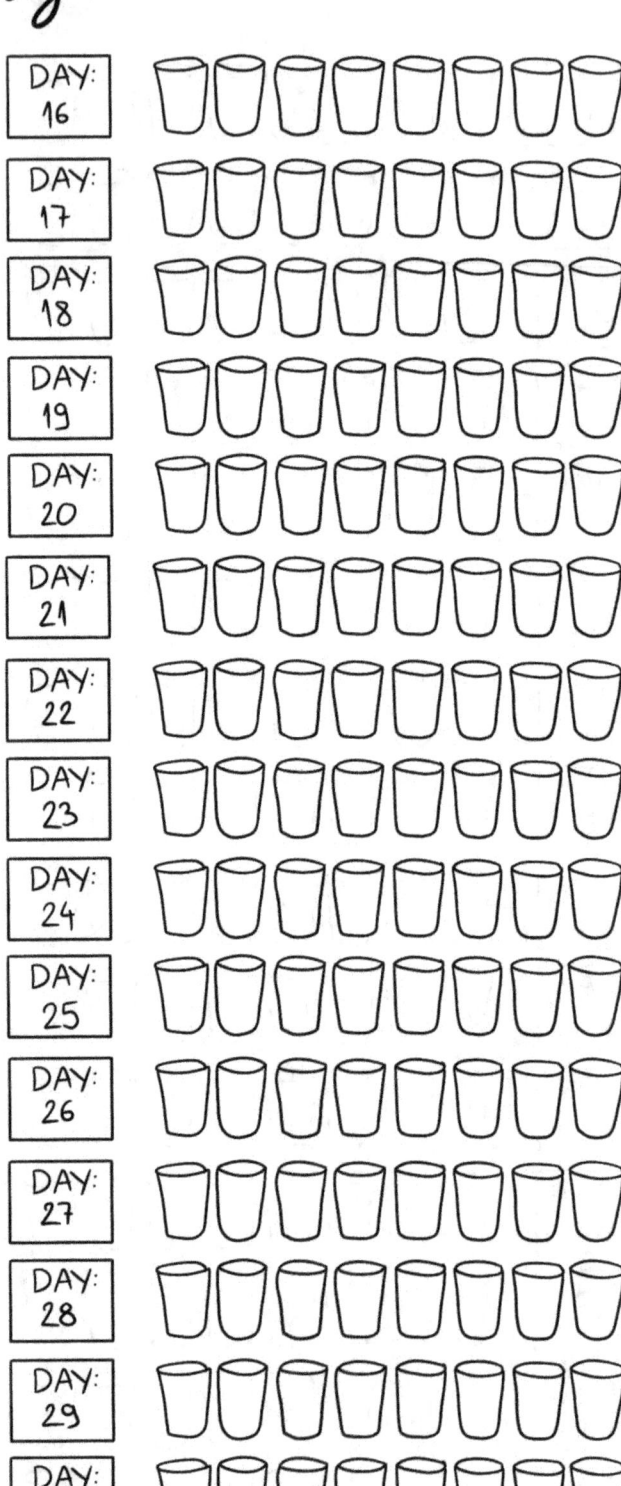

30 DAY WATER challenge

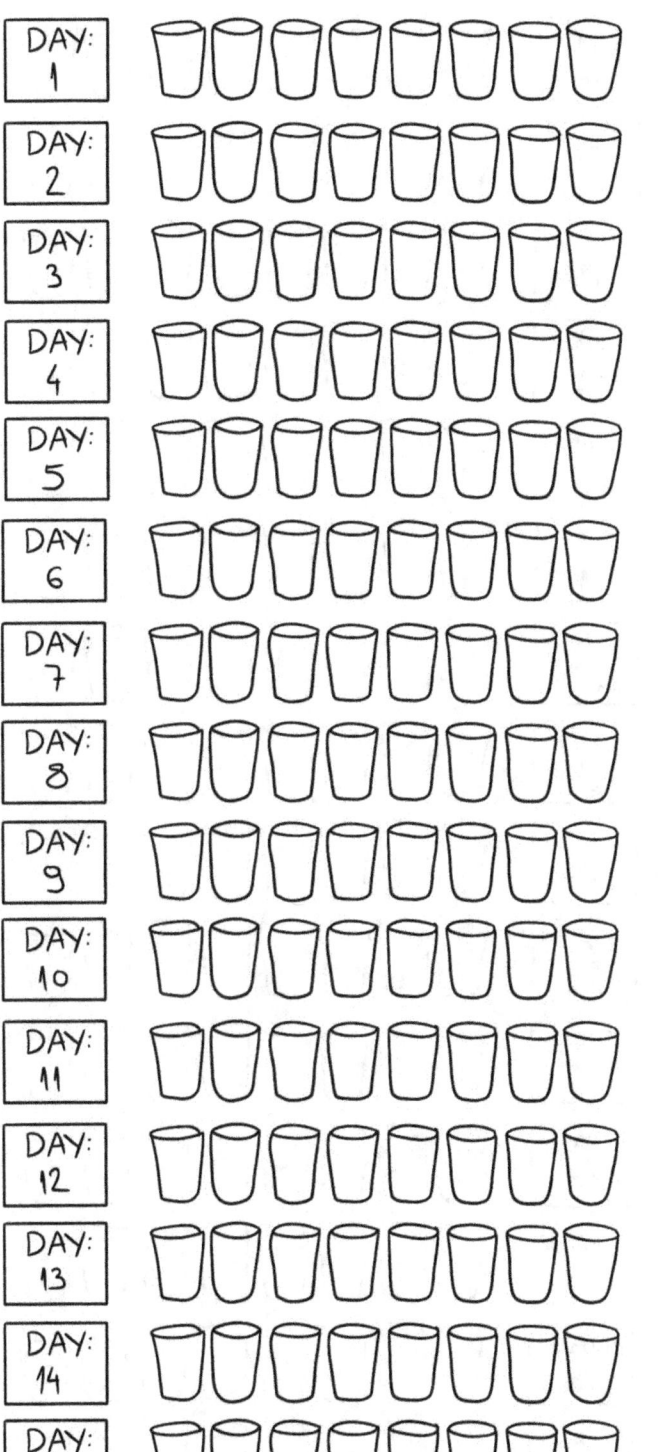

DAY:								
1	▢	▢	▢	▢	▢	▢	▢	▢
2	▢	▢	▢	▢	▢	▢	▢	▢
3	▢	▢	▢	▢	▢	▢	▢	▢
4	▢	▢	▢	▢	▢	▢	▢	▢
5	▢	▢	▢	▢	▢	▢	▢	▢
6	▢	▢	▢	▢	▢	▢	▢	▢
7	▢	▢	▢	▢	▢	▢	▢	▢
8	▢	▢	▢	▢	▢	▢	▢	▢
9	▢	▢	▢	▢	▢	▢	▢	▢
10	▢	▢	▢	▢	▢	▢	▢	▢
11	▢	▢	▢	▢	▢	▢	▢	▢
12	▢	▢	▢	▢	▢	▢	▢	▢
13	▢	▢	▢	▢	▢	▢	▢	▢
14	▢	▢	▢	▢	▢	▢	▢	▢
15	▢	▢	▢	▢	▢	▢	▢	▢

DAY:								
16	▢	▢	▢	▢	▢	▢	▢	▢
17	▢	▢	▢	▢	▢	▢	▢	▢
18	▢	▢	▢	▢	▢	▢	▢	▢
19	▢	▢	▢	▢	▢	▢	▢	▢
20	▢	▢	▢	▢	▢	▢	▢	▢
21	▢	▢	▢	▢	▢	▢	▢	▢
22	▢	▢	▢	▢	▢	▢	▢	▢
23	▢	▢	▢	▢	▢	▢	▢	▢
24	▢	▢	▢	▢	▢	▢	▢	▢
25	▢	▢	▢	▢	▢	▢	▢	▢
26	▢	▢	▢	▢	▢	▢	▢	▢
27	▢	▢	▢	▢	▢	▢	▢	▢
28	▢	▢	▢	▢	▢	▢	▢	▢
29	▢	▢	▢	▢	▢	▢	▢	▢
30	▢	▢	▢	▢	▢	▢	▢	▢

30 DAY
WATER
challenge

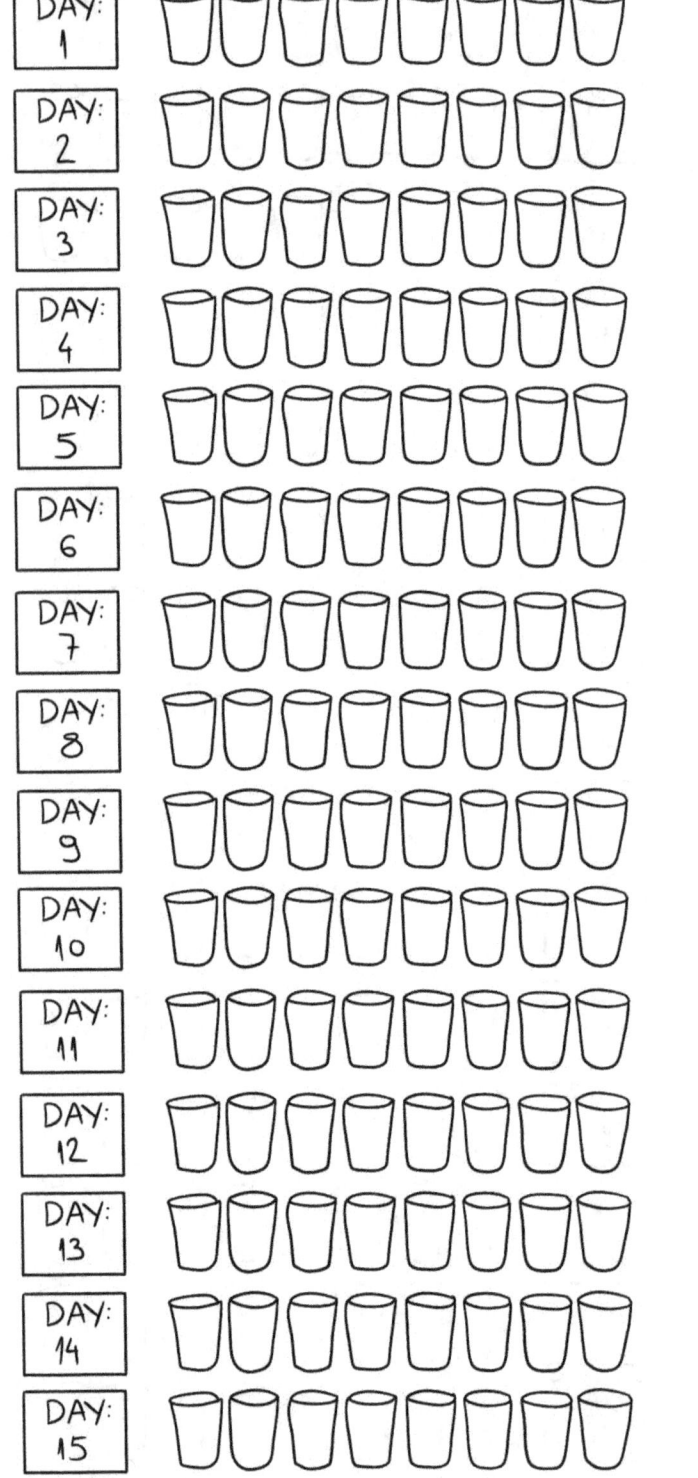

DAY: 1	DAY: 16
DAY: 2	DAY: 17
DAY: 3	DAY: 18
DAY: 4	DAY: 19
DAY: 5	DAY: 20
DAY: 6	DAY: 21
DAY: 7	DAY: 22
DAY: 8	DAY: 23
DAY: 9	DAY: 24
DAY: 10	DAY: 25
DAY: 11	DAY: 26
DAY: 12	DAY: 27
DAY: 13	DAY: 28
DAY: 14	DAY: 29
DAY: 15	DAY: 30

30 DAY
WATER
challenge

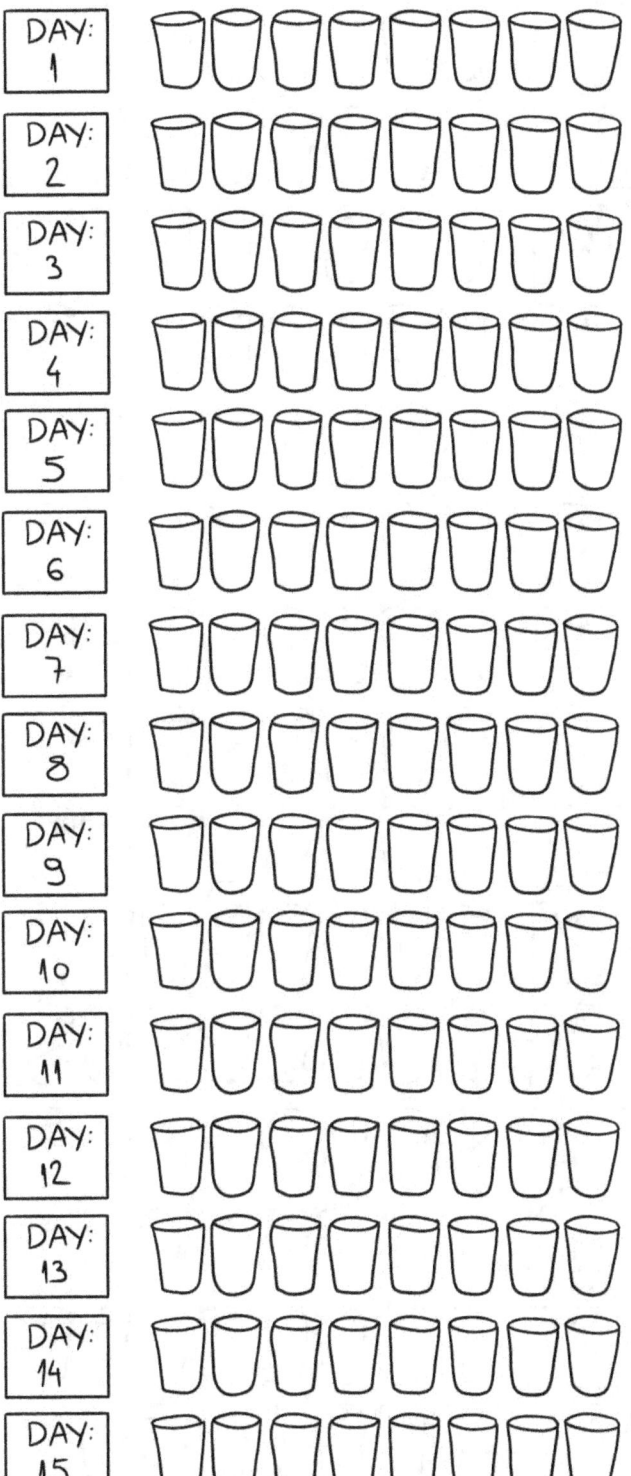

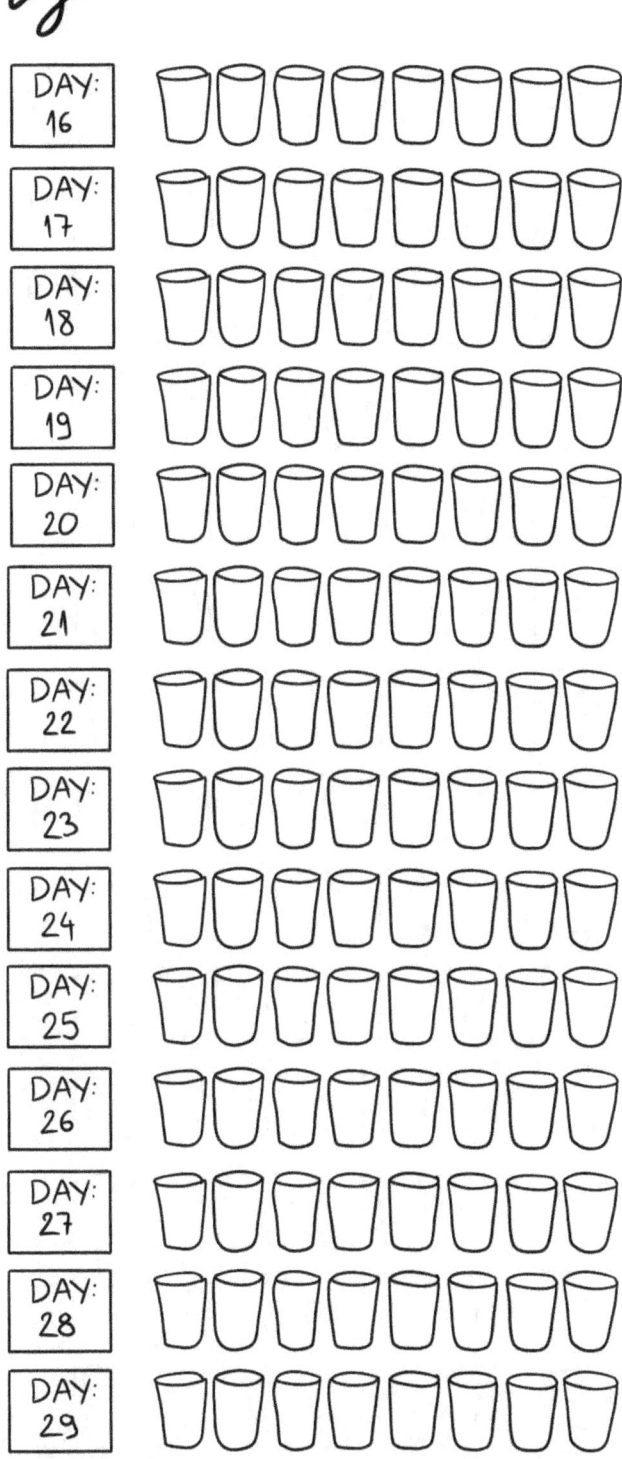

30 DAY
WATER
challenge

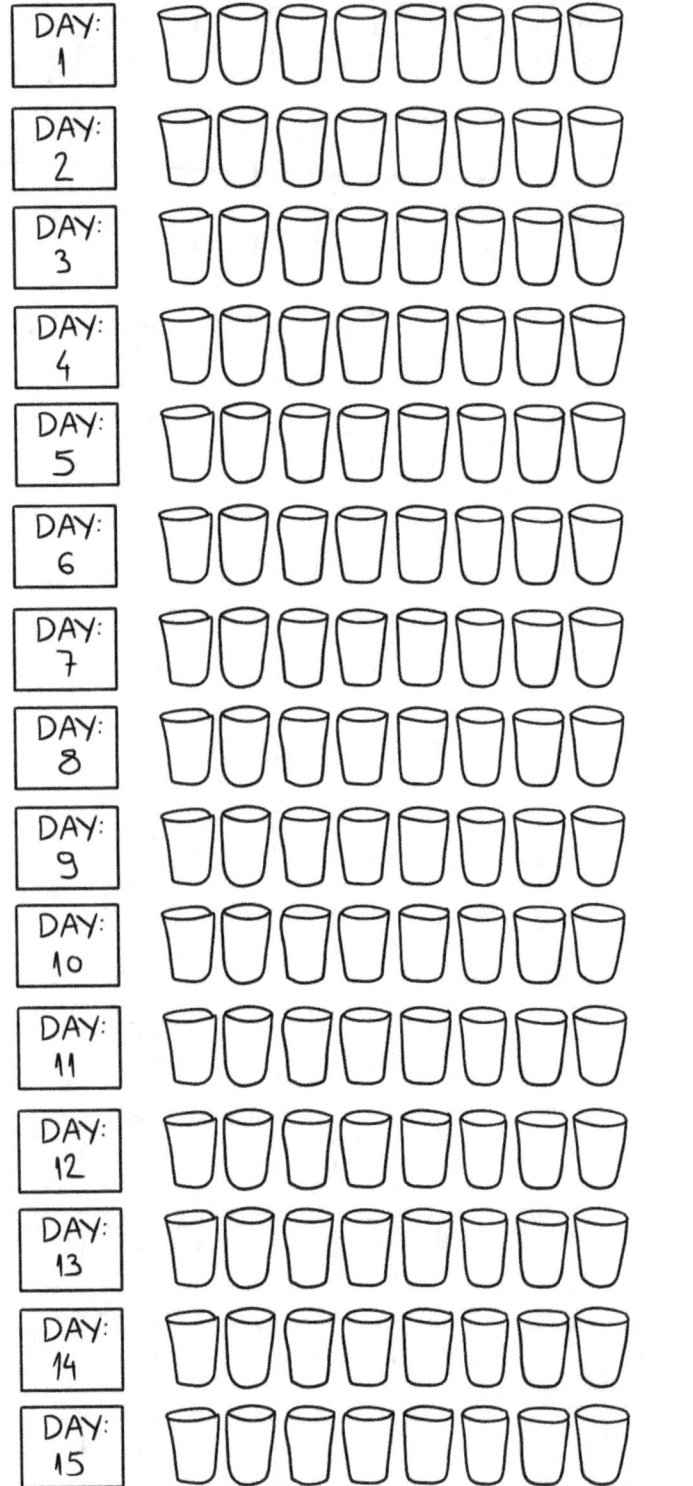

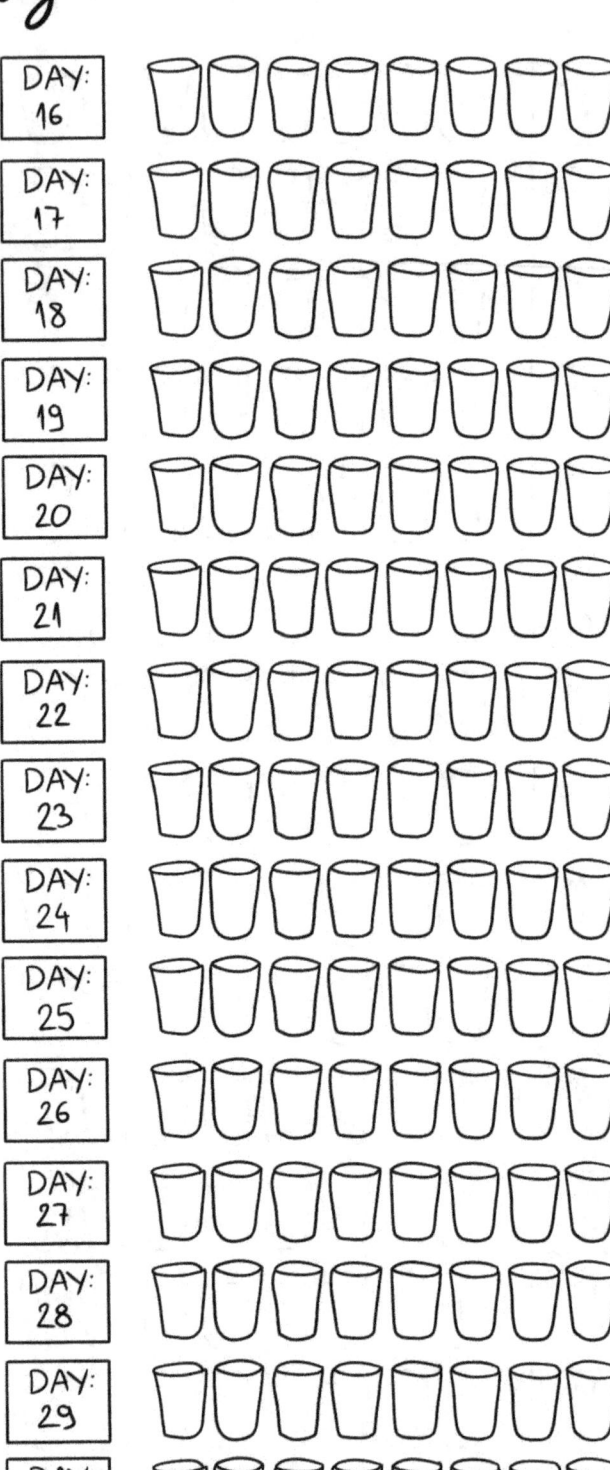

30 DAY
WATER
challenge

DAY: 1	🥤🥤🥤🥤🥤🥤🥤🥤	DAY: 16	🥤🥤🥤🥤🥤🥤🥤🥤
DAY: 2	🥤🥤🥤🥤🥤🥤🥤🥤	DAY: 17	🥤🥤🥤🥤🥤🥤🥤🥤
DAY: 3	🥤🥤🥤🥤🥤🥤🥤🥤	DAY: 18	🥤🥤🥤🥤🥤🥤🥤🥤
DAY: 4	🥤🥤🥤🥤🥤🥤🥤🥤	DAY: 19	🥤🥤🥤🥤🥤🥤🥤🥤
DAY: 5	🥤🥤🥤🥤🥤🥤🥤🥤	DAY: 20	🥤🥤🥤🥤🥤🥤🥤🥤
DAY: 6	🥤🥤🥤🥤🥤🥤🥤🥤	DAY: 21	🥤🥤🥤🥤🥤🥤🥤🥤
DAY: 7	🥤🥤🥤🥤🥤🥤🥤🥤	DAY: 22	🥤🥤🥤🥤🥤🥤🥤🥤
DAY: 8	🥤🥤🥤🥤🥤🥤🥤🥤	DAY: 23	🥤🥤🥤🥤🥤🥤🥤🥤
DAY: 9	🥤🥤🥤🥤🥤🥤🥤🥤	DAY: 24	🥤🥤🥤🥤🥤🥤🥤🥤
DAY: 10	🥤🥤🥤🥤🥤🥤🥤🥤	DAY: 25	🥤🥤🥤🥤🥤🥤🥤🥤
DAY: 11	🥤🥤🥤🥤🥤🥤🥤🥤	DAY: 26	🥤🥤🥤🥤🥤🥤🥤🥤
DAY: 12	🥤🥤🥤🥤🥤🥤🥤🥤	DAY: 27	🥤🥤🥤🥤🥤🥤🥤🥤
DAY: 13	🥤🥤🥤🥤🥤🥤🥤🥤	DAY: 28	🥤🥤🥤🥤🥤🥤🥤🥤
DAY: 14	🥤🥤🥤🥤🥤🥤🥤🥤	DAY: 29	🥤🥤🥤🥤🥤🥤🥤🥤
DAY: 15	🥤🥤🥤🥤🥤🥤🥤🥤	DAY: 30	🥤🥤🥤🥤🥤🥤🥤🥤

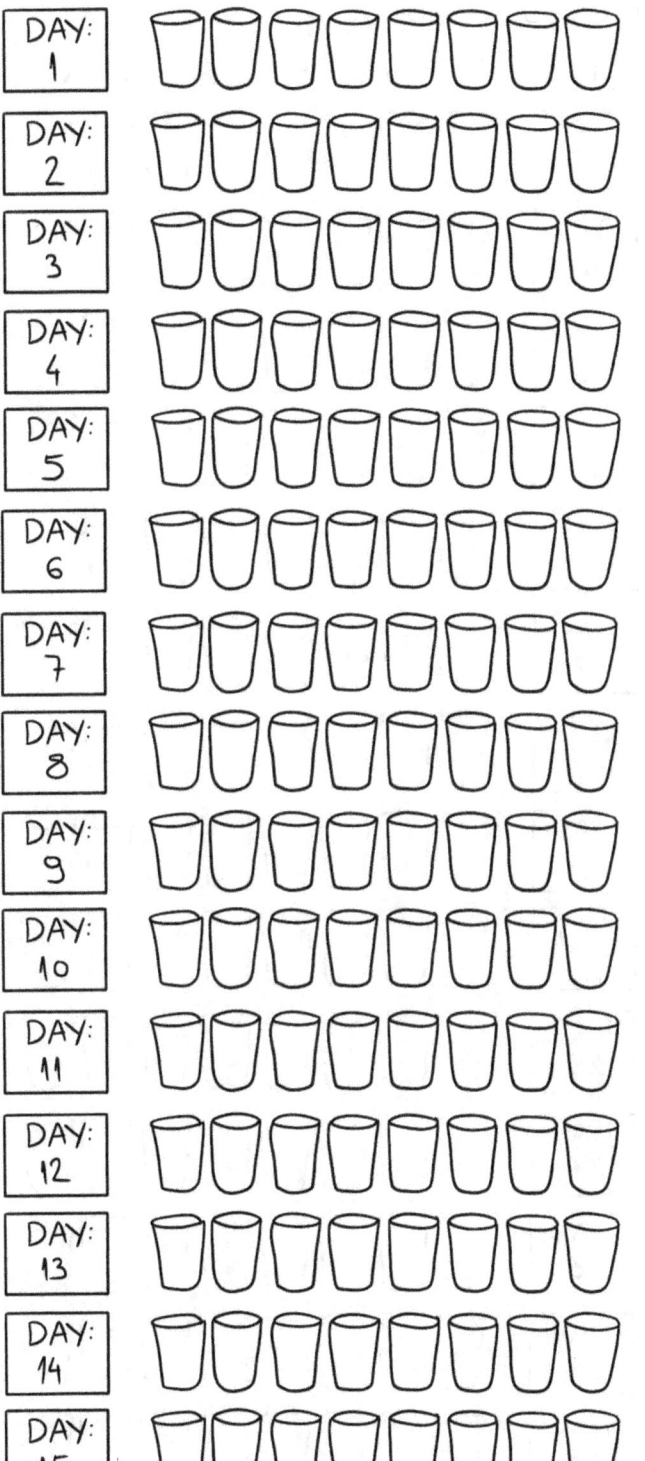

30 DAY
WATER
challenge

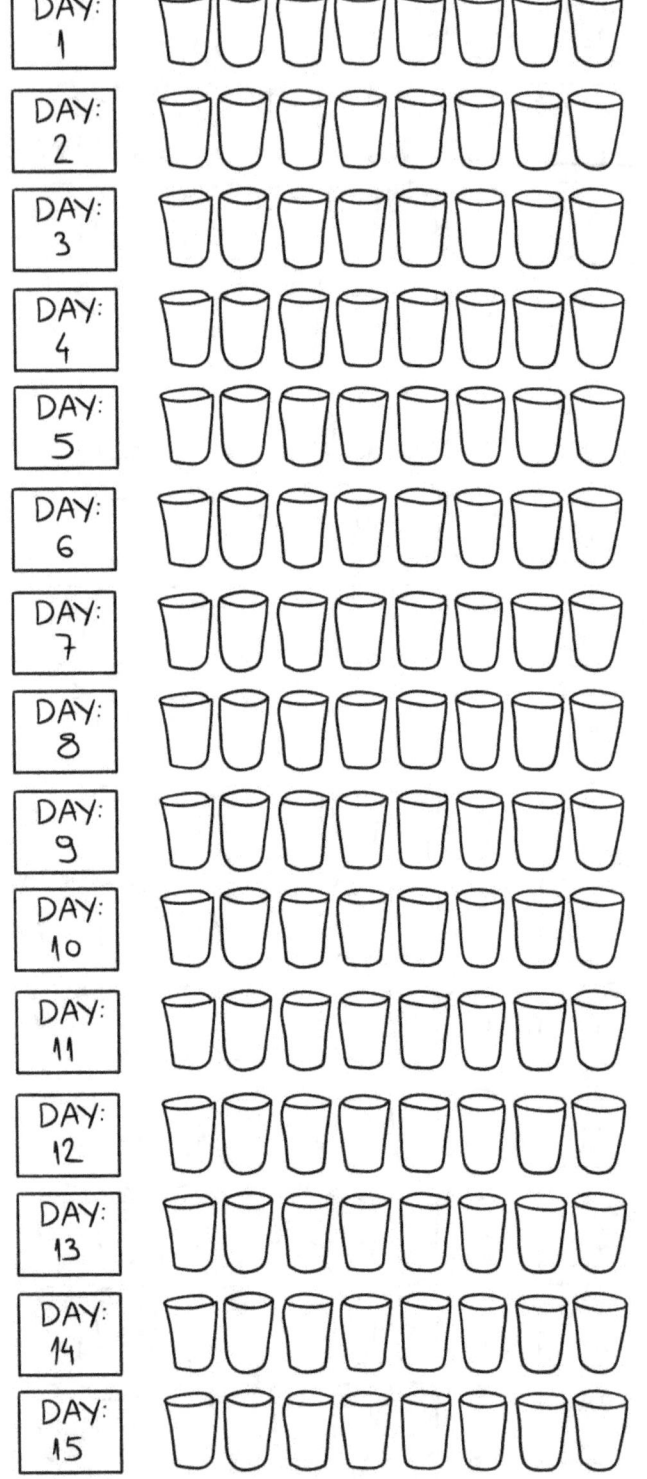

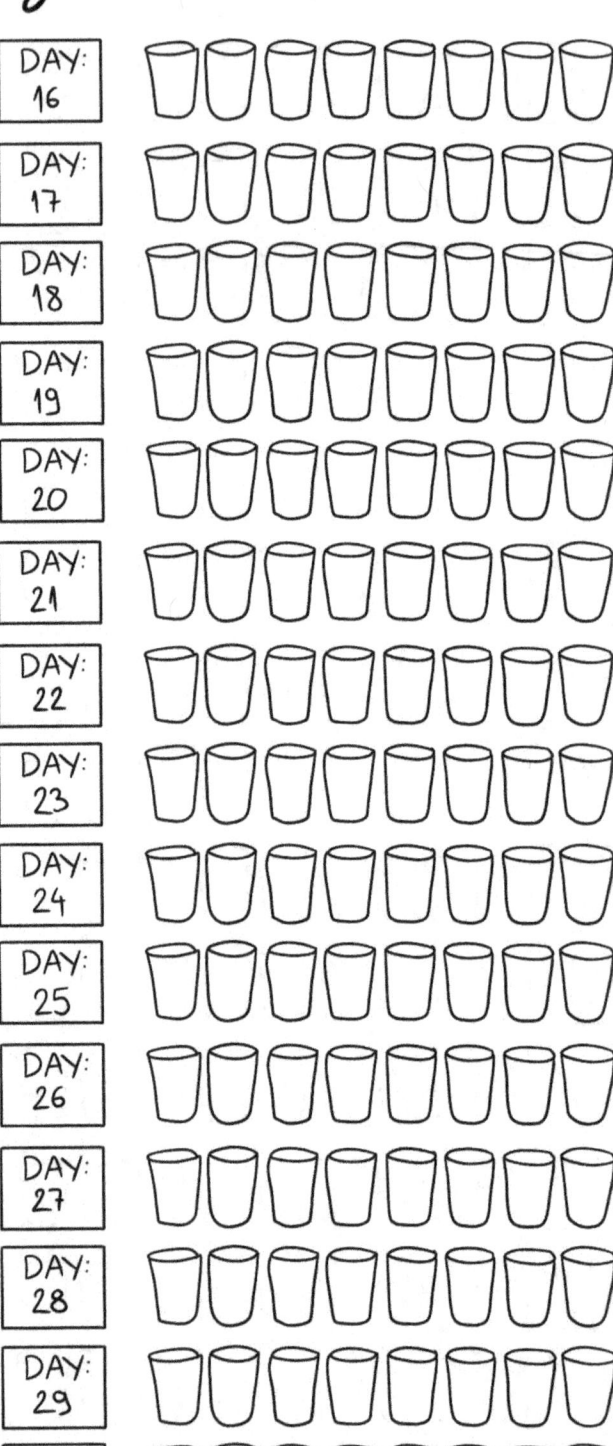

30 DAY
WATER
challenge

DAY: 1	🥤🥤🥤🥤🥤🥤🥤🥤
DAY: 2	🥤🥤🥤🥤🥤🥤🥤🥤
DAY: 3	🥤🥤🥤🥤🥤🥤🥤🥤
DAY: 4	🥤🥤🥤🥤🥤🥤🥤🥤
DAY: 5	🥤🥤🥤🥤🥤🥤🥤🥤
DAY: 6	🥤🥤🥤🥤🥤🥤🥤🥤
DAY: 7	🥤🥤🥤🥤🥤🥤🥤🥤
DAY: 8	🥤🥤🥤🥤🥤🥤🥤🥤
DAY: 9	🥤🥤🥤🥤🥤🥤🥤🥤
DAY: 10	🥤🥤🥤🥤🥤🥤🥤🥤
DAY: 11	🥤🥤🥤🥤🥤🥤🥤🥤
DAY: 12	🥤🥤🥤🥤🥤🥤🥤🥤
DAY: 13	🥤🥤🥤🥤🥤🥤🥤🥤
DAY: 14	🥤🥤🥤🥤🥤🥤🥤🥤
DAY: 15	🥤🥤🥤🥤🥤🥤🥤🥤
DAY: 16	🥤🥤🥤🥤🥤🥤🥤🥤
DAY: 17	🥤🥤🥤🥤🥤🥤🥤🥤
DAY: 18	🥤🥤🥤🥤🥤🥤🥤🥤
DAY: 19	🥤🥤🥤🥤🥤🥤🥤🥤
DAY: 20	🥤🥤🥤🥤🥤🥤🥤🥤
DAY: 21	🥤🥤🥤🥤🥤🥤🥤🥤
DAY: 22	🥤🥤🥤🥤🥤🥤🥤🥤
DAY: 23	🥤🥤🥤🥤🥤🥤🥤🥤
DAY: 24	🥤🥤🥤🥤🥤🥤🥤🥤
DAY: 25	🥤🥤🥤🥤🥤🥤🥤🥤
DAY: 26	🥤🥤🥤🥤🥤🥤🥤🥤
DAY: 27	🥤🥤🥤🥤🥤🥤🥤🥤
DAY: 28	🥤🥤🥤🥤🥤🥤🥤🥤
DAY: 29	🥤🥤🥤🥤🥤🥤🥤🥤
DAY: 30	🥤🥤🥤🥤🥤🥤🥤🥤

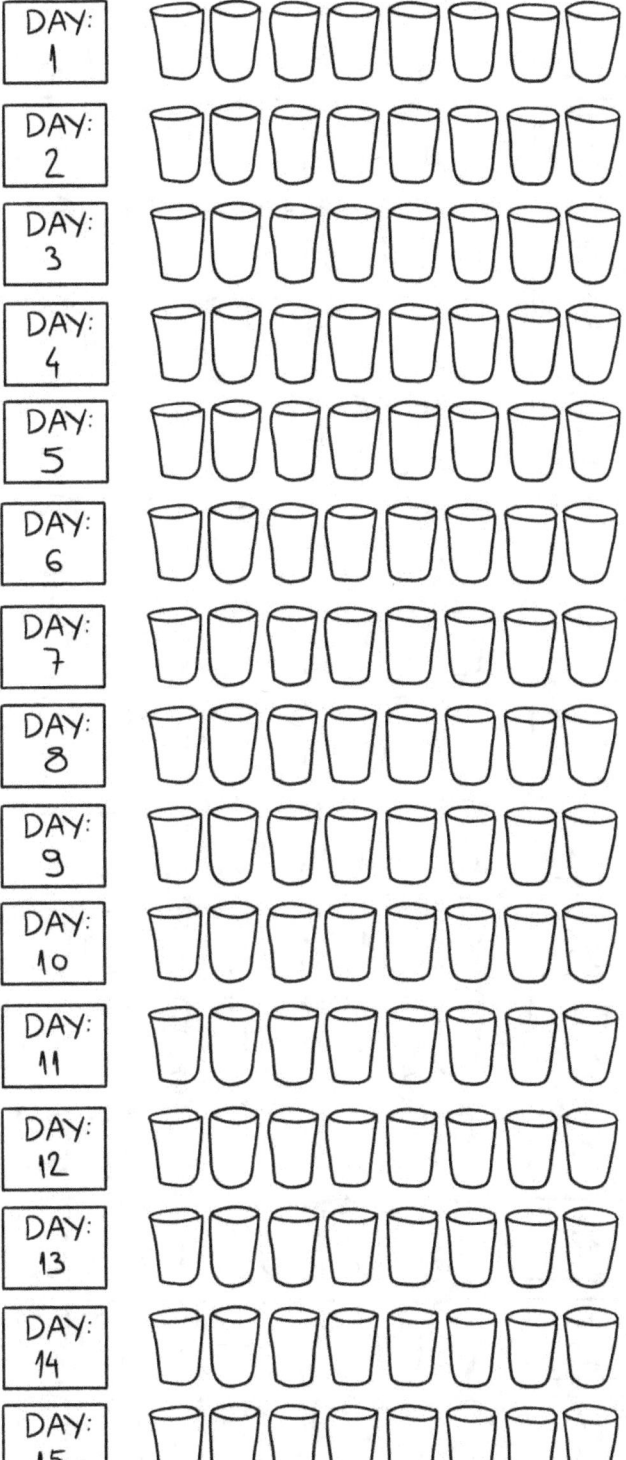

30 DAY WATER challenge

DAY: 1	🥛🥛🥛🥛🥛🥛🥛🥛
DAY: 2	🥛🥛🥛🥛🥛🥛🥛🥛
DAY: 3	🥛🥛🥛🥛🥛🥛🥛🥛
DAY: 4	🥛🥛🥛🥛🥛🥛🥛🥛
DAY: 5	🥛🥛🥛🥛🥛🥛🥛🥛
DAY: 6	🥛🥛🥛🥛🥛🥛🥛🥛
DAY: 7	🥛🥛🥛🥛🥛🥛🥛🥛
DAY: 8	🥛🥛🥛🥛🥛🥛🥛🥛
DAY: 9	🥛🥛🥛🥛🥛🥛🥛🥛
DAY: 10	🥛🥛🥛🥛🥛🥛🥛🥛
DAY: 11	🥛🥛🥛🥛🥛🥛🥛🥛
DAY: 12	🥛🥛🥛🥛🥛🥛🥛🥛
DAY: 13	🥛🥛🥛🥛🥛🥛🥛🥛
DAY: 14	🥛🥛🥛🥛🥛🥛🥛🥛
DAY: 15	🥛🥛🥛🥛🥛🥛🥛🥛

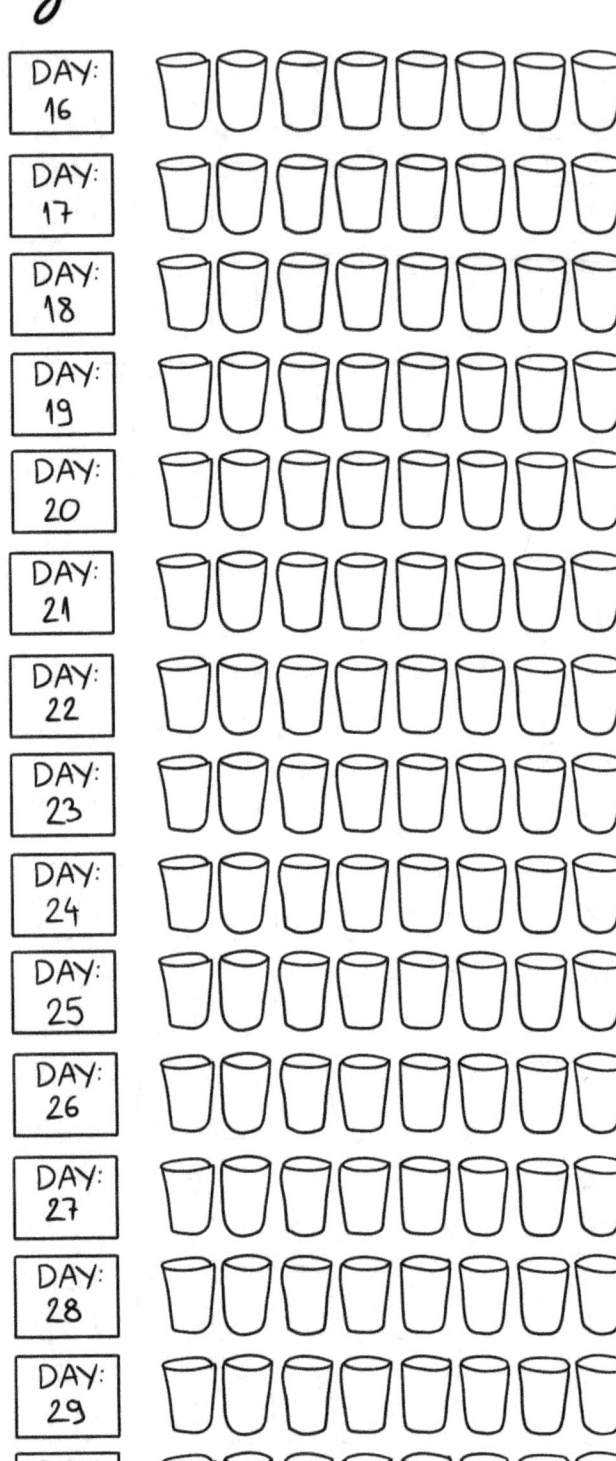

DAY: 16	🥛🥛🥛🥛🥛🥛🥛🥛
DAY: 17	🥛🥛🥛🥛🥛🥛🥛🥛
DAY: 18	🥛🥛🥛🥛🥛🥛🥛🥛
DAY: 19	🥛🥛🥛🥛🥛🥛🥛🥛
DAY: 20	🥛🥛🥛🥛🥛🥛🥛🥛
DAY: 21	🥛🥛🥛🥛🥛🥛🥛🥛
DAY: 22	🥛🥛🥛🥛🥛🥛🥛🥛
DAY: 23	🥛🥛🥛🥛🥛🥛🥛🥛
DAY: 24	🥛🥛🥛🥛🥛🥛🥛🥛
DAY: 25	🥛🥛🥛🥛🥛🥛🥛🥛
DAY: 26	🥛🥛🥛🥛🥛🥛🥛🥛
DAY: 27	🥛🥛🥛🥛🥛🥛🥛🥛
DAY: 28	🥛🥛🥛🥛🥛🥛🥛🥛
DAY: 29	🥛🥛🥛🥛🥛🥛🥛🥛
DAY: 30	🥛🥛🥛🥛🥛🥛🥛🥛

30 DAY
WATER
challenge

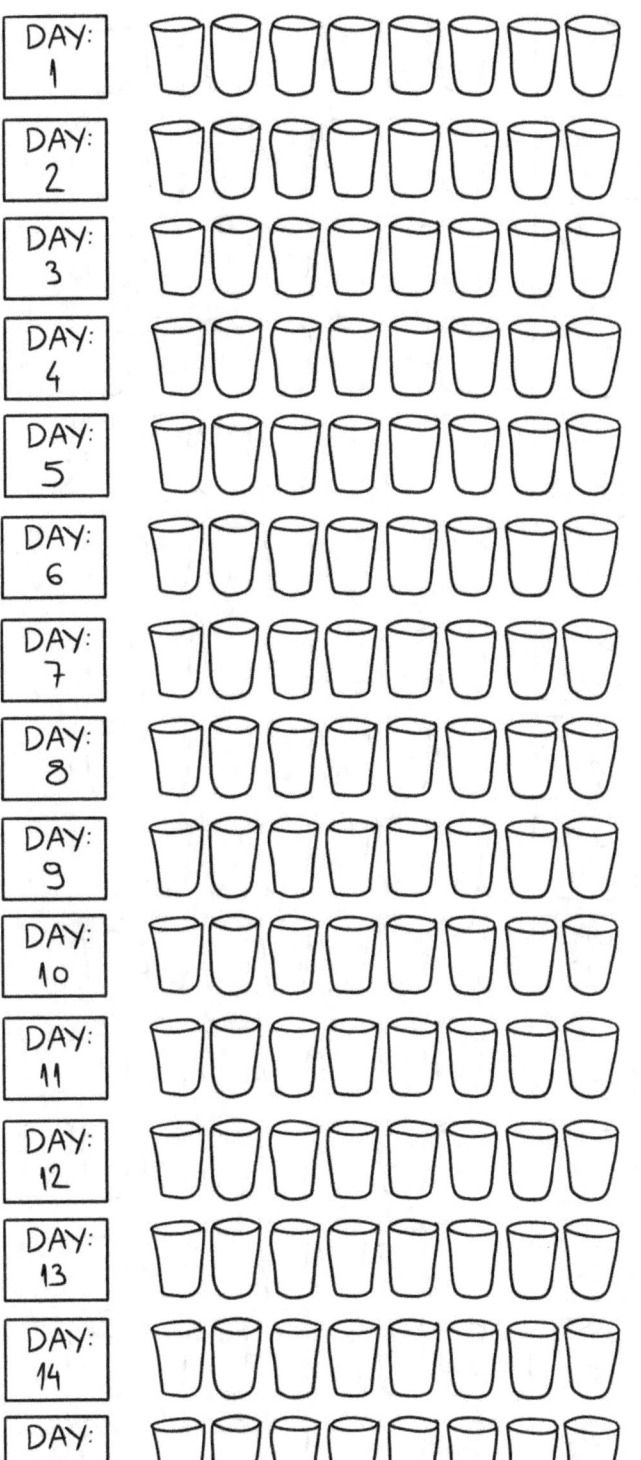

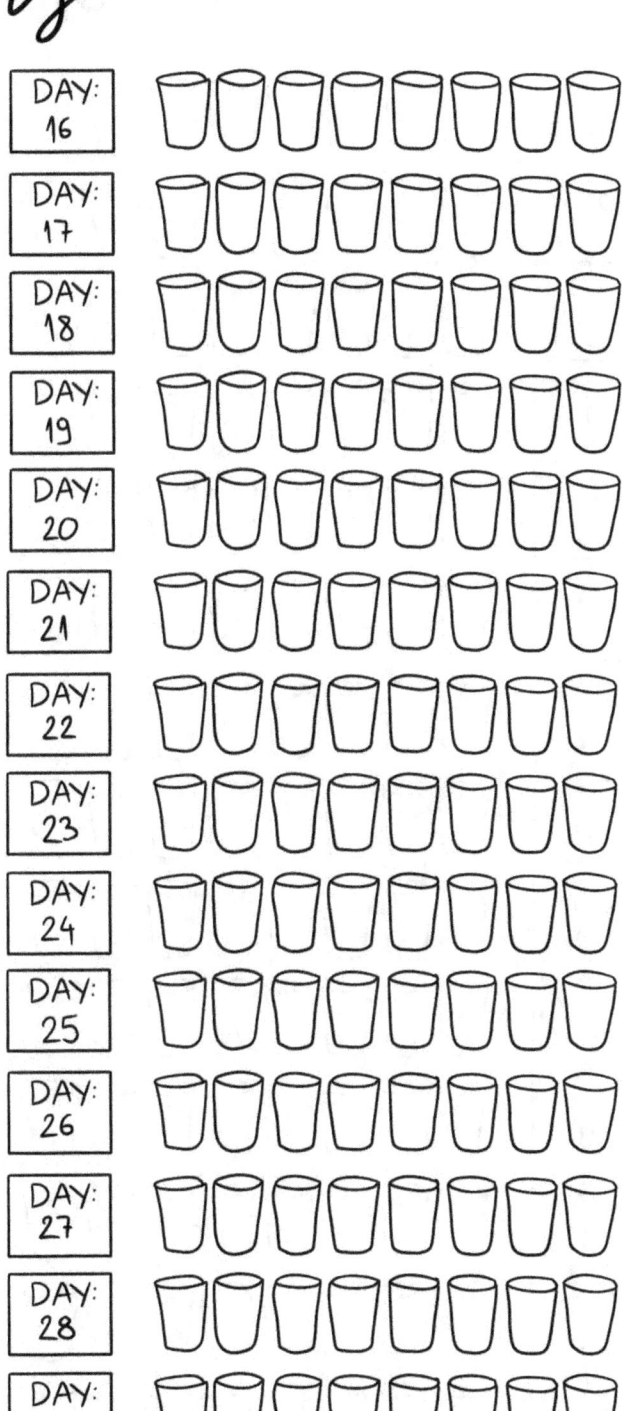

30 DAY
WATER
challenge

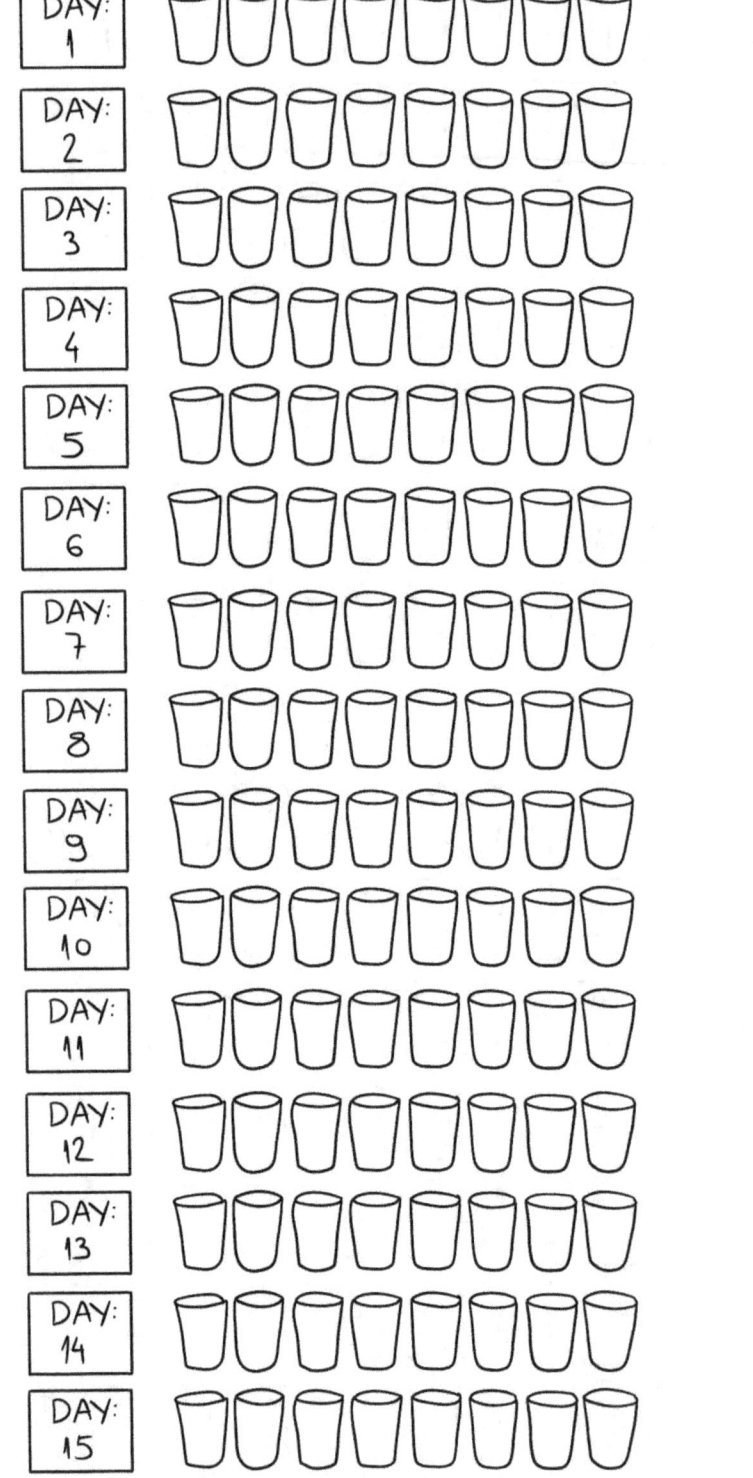

DAY: 1	DAY: 16
DAY: 2	DAY: 17
DAY: 3	DAY: 18
DAY: 4	DAY: 19
DAY: 5	DAY: 20
DAY: 6	DAY: 21
DAY: 7	DAY: 22
DAY: 8	DAY: 23
DAY: 9	DAY: 24
DAY: 10	DAY: 25
DAY: 11	DAY: 26
DAY: 12	DAY: 27
DAY: 13	DAY: 28
DAY: 14	DAY: 29
DAY: 15	DAY: 30

30 DAY
WATER
challenge

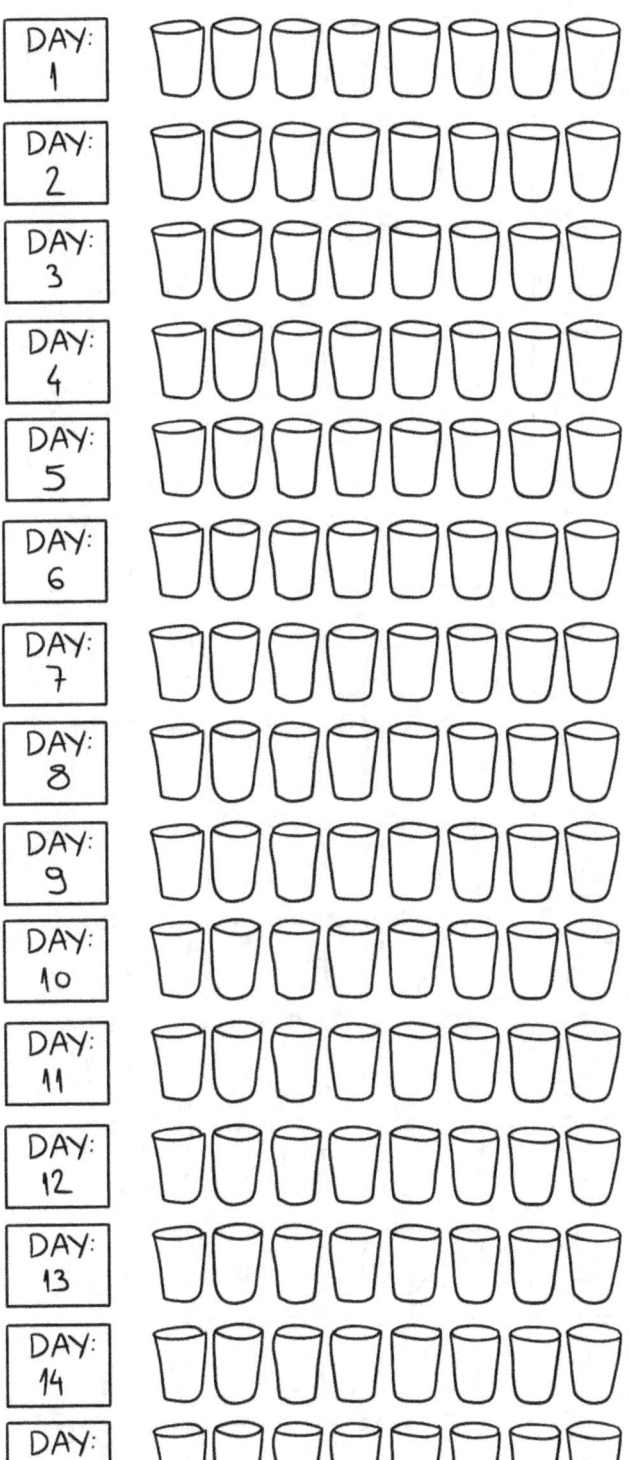

DAY: 1								
DAY: 2								
DAY: 3								
DAY: 4								
DAY: 5								
DAY: 6								
DAY: 7								
DAY: 8								
DAY: 9								
DAY: 10								
DAY: 11								
DAY: 12								
DAY: 13								
DAY: 14								
DAY: 15								

DAY: 16								
DAY: 17								
DAY: 18								
DAY: 19								
DAY: 20								
DAY: 21								
DAY: 22								
DAY: 23								
DAY: 24								
DAY: 25								
DAY: 26								
DAY: 27								
DAY: 28								
DAY: 29								
DAY: 30								

30 DAY
WATER
challenge

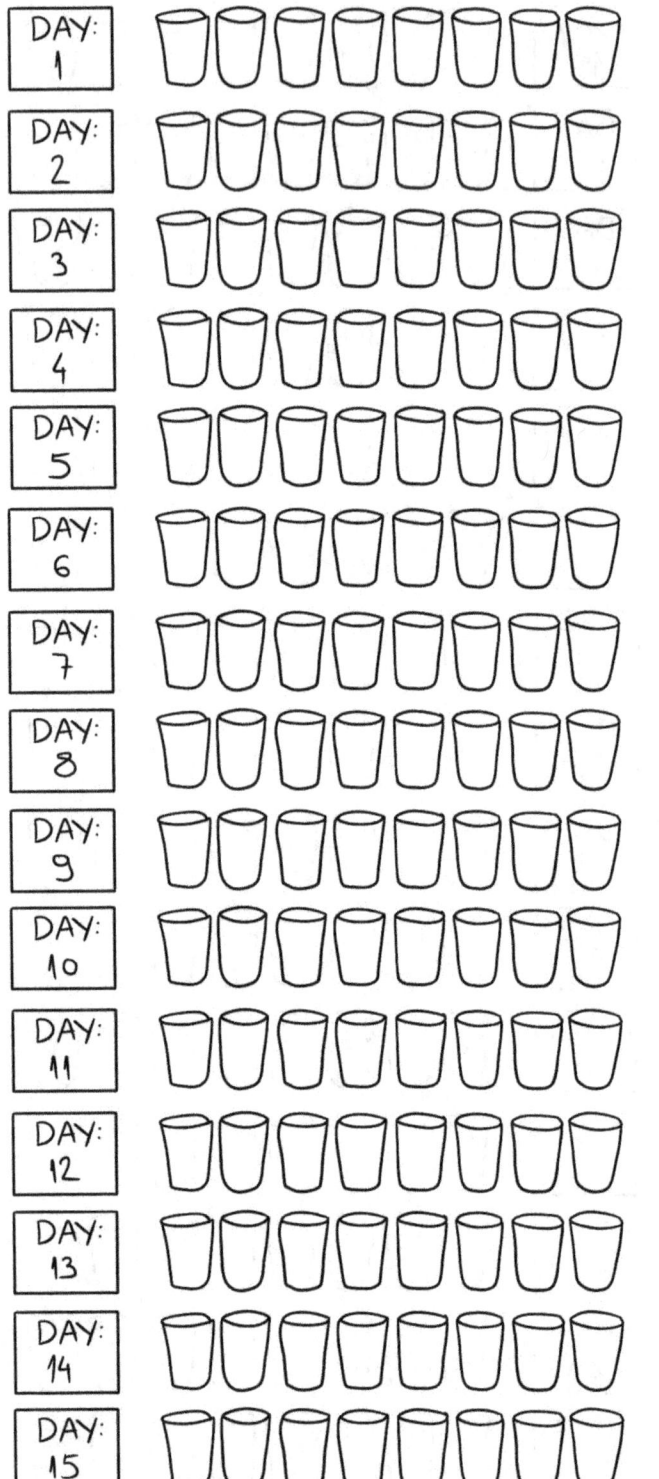

DAY: 1							
DAY: 2							
DAY: 3							
DAY: 4							
DAY: 5							
DAY: 6							
DAY: 7							
DAY: 8							
DAY: 9							
DAY: 10							
DAY: 11							
DAY: 12							
DAY: 13							
DAY: 14							
DAY: 15							

DAY: 16							
DAY: 17							
DAY: 18							
DAY: 19							
DAY: 20							
DAY: 21							
DAY: 22							
DAY: 23							
DAY: 24							
DAY: 25							
DAY: 26							
DAY: 27							
DAY: 28							
DAY: 29							
DAY: 30							

30 DAY
WATER
challenge

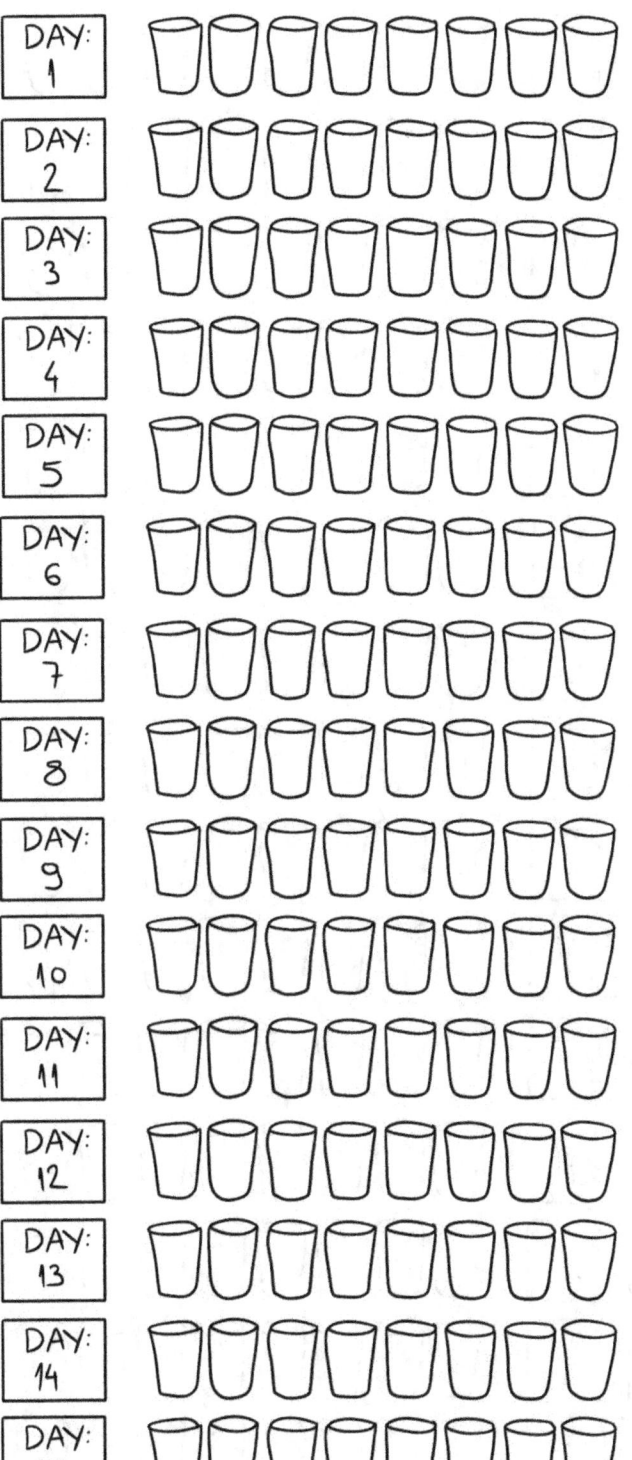

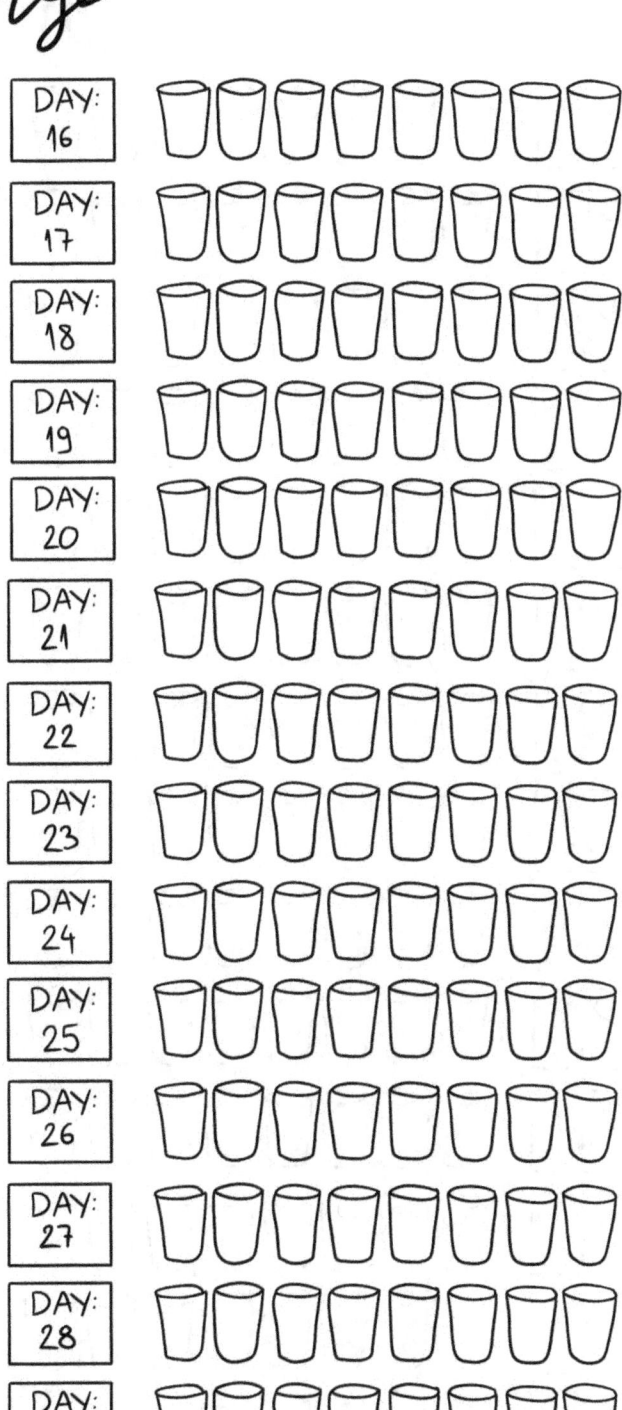

30 DAY
WATER
challenge

DAY: 1	ᵁᵁᵁᵁᵁᵁᵁᵁ	DAY: 16	ᵁᵁᵁᵁᵁᵁᵁᵁ
DAY: 2	ᵁᵁᵁᵁᵁᵁᵁᵁ	DAY: 17	ᵁᵁᵁᵁᵁᵁᵁᵁ
DAY: 3	ᵁᵁᵁᵁᵁᵁᵁᵁ	DAY: 18	ᵁᵁᵁᵁᵁᵁᵁᵁ
DAY: 4	ᵁᵁᵁᵁᵁᵁᵁᵁ	DAY: 19	ᵁᵁᵁᵁᵁᵁᵁᵁ
DAY: 5	ᵁᵁᵁᵁᵁᵁᵁᵁ	DAY: 20	ᵁᵁᵁᵁᵁᵁᵁᵁ
DAY: 6	ᵁᵁᵁᵁᵁᵁᵁᵁ	DAY: 21	ᵁᵁᵁᵁᵁᵁᵁᵁ
DAY: 7	ᵁᵁᵁᵁᵁᵁᵁᵁ	DAY: 22	ᵁᵁᵁᵁᵁᵁᵁᵁ
DAY: 8	ᵁᵁᵁᵁᵁᵁᵁᵁ	DAY: 23	ᵁᵁᵁᵁᵁᵁᵁᵁ
DAY: 9	ᵁᵁᵁᵁᵁᵁᵁᵁ	DAY: 24	ᵁᵁᵁᵁᵁᵁᵁᵁ
DAY: 10	ᵁᵁᵁᵁᵁᵁᵁᵁ	DAY: 25	ᵁᵁᵁᵁᵁᵁᵁᵁ
DAY: 11	ᵁᵁᵁᵁᵁᵁᵁᵁ	DAY: 26	ᵁᵁᵁᵁᵁᵁᵁᵁ
DAY: 12	ᵁᵁᵁᵁᵁᵁᵁᵁ	DAY: 27	ᵁᵁᵁᵁᵁᵁᵁᵁ
DAY: 13	ᵁᵁᵁᵁᵁᵁᵁᵁ	DAY: 28	ᵁᵁᵁᵁᵁᵁᵁᵁ
DAY: 14	ᵁᵁᵁᵁᵁᵁᵁᵁ	DAY: 29	ᵁᵁᵁᵁᵁᵁᵁᵁ
DAY: 15	ᵁᵁᵁᵁᵁᵁᵁᵁ	DAY: 30	ᵁᵁᵁᵁᵁᵁᵁᵁ

30 DAY
WATER
challenge

DAY: 1	DAY: 16
DAY: 2	DAY: 17
DAY: 3	DAY: 18
DAY: 4	DAY: 19
DAY: 5	DAY: 20
DAY: 6	DAY: 21
DAY: 7	DAY: 22
DAY: 8	DAY: 23
DAY: 9	DAY: 24
DAY: 10	DAY: 25
DAY: 11	DAY: 26
DAY: 12	DAY: 27
DAY: 13	DAY: 28
DAY: 14	DAY: 29
DAY: 15	DAY: 30

30 DAY
WATER
challenge

DAY: 1								
DAY: 2								
DAY: 3								
DAY: 4								
DAY: 5								
DAY: 6								
DAY: 7								
DAY: 8								
DAY: 9								
DAY: 10								
DAY: 11								
DAY: 12								
DAY: 13								
DAY: 14								
DAY: 15								

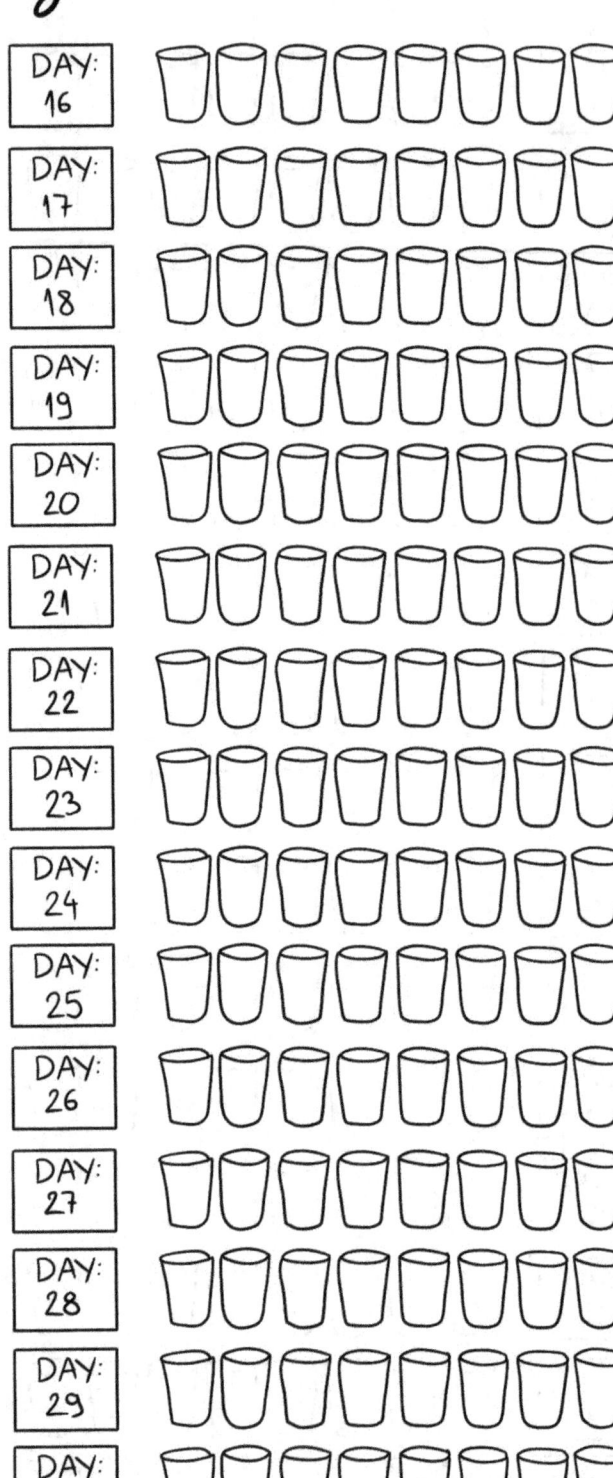

DAY: 16								
DAY: 17								
DAY: 18								
DAY: 19								
DAY: 20								
DAY: 21								
DAY: 22								
DAY: 23								
DAY: 24								
DAY: 25								
DAY: 26								
DAY: 27								
DAY: 28								
DAY: 29								
DAY: 30								

30 DAY
WATER
challenge

DAY: 1	DAY: 16	
DAY: 2	DAY: 17	
DAY: 3	DAY: 18	
DAY: 4	DAY: 19	
DAY: 5	DAY: 20	
DAY: 6	DAY: 21	
DAY: 7	DAY: 22	
DAY: 8	DAY: 23	
DAY: 9	DAY: 24	
DAY: 10	DAY: 25	
DAY: 11	DAY: 26	
DAY: 12	DAY: 27	
DAY: 13	DAY: 28	
DAY: 14	DAY: 29	
DAY: 15	DAY: 30	

30 DAY
WATER
challenge

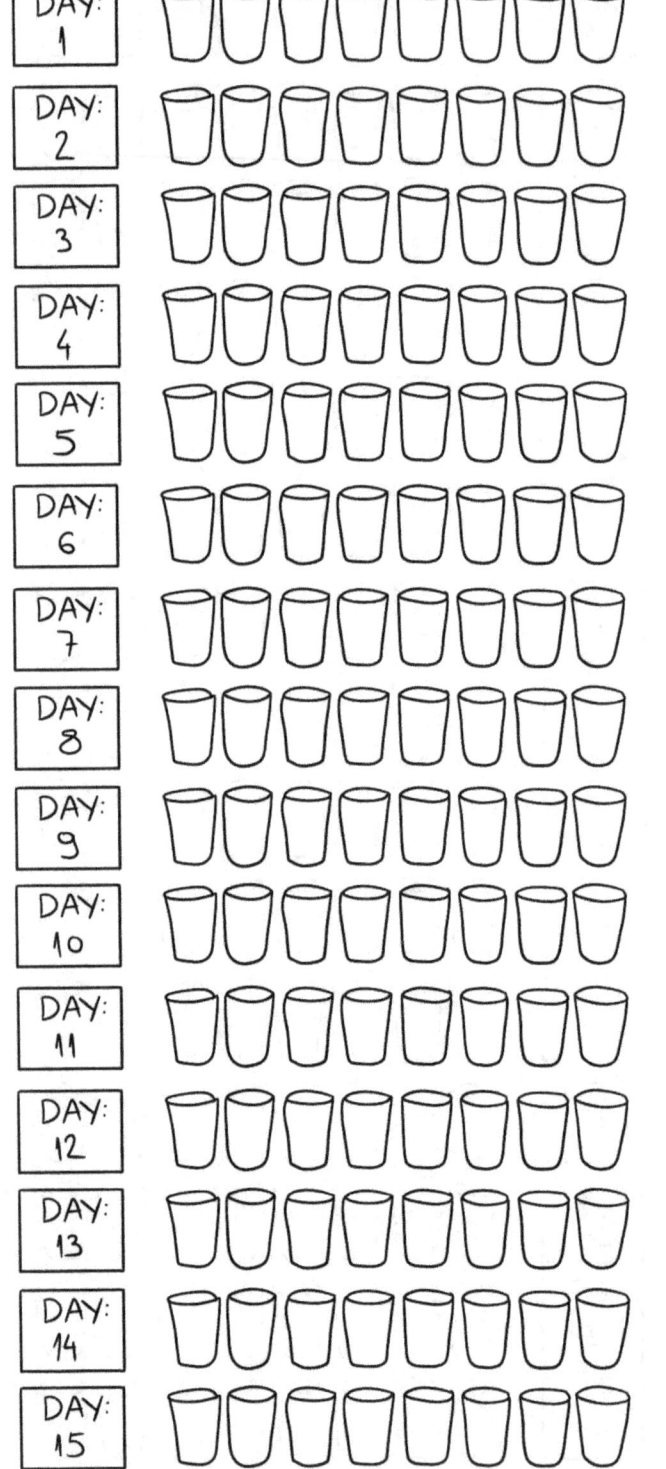

DAY: 1	⊔⊔⊔⊔⊔⊔⊔⊔
DAY: 2	⊔⊔⊔⊔⊔⊔⊔⊔
DAY: 3	⊔⊔⊔⊔⊔⊔⊔⊔
DAY: 4	⊔⊔⊔⊔⊔⊔⊔⊔
DAY: 5	⊔⊔⊔⊔⊔⊔⊔⊔
DAY: 6	⊔⊔⊔⊔⊔⊔⊔⊔
DAY: 7	⊔⊔⊔⊔⊔⊔⊔⊔
DAY: 8	⊔⊔⊔⊔⊔⊔⊔⊔
DAY: 9	⊔⊔⊔⊔⊔⊔⊔⊔
DAY: 10	⊔⊔⊔⊔⊔⊔⊔⊔
DAY: 11	⊔⊔⊔⊔⊔⊔⊔⊔
DAY: 12	⊔⊔⊔⊔⊔⊔⊔⊔
DAY: 13	⊔⊔⊔⊔⊔⊔⊔⊔
DAY: 14	⊔⊔⊔⊔⊔⊔⊔⊔
DAY: 15	⊔⊔⊔⊔⊔⊔⊔⊔

DAY: 16	⊔⊔⊔⊔⊔⊔⊔⊔
DAY: 17	⊔⊔⊔⊔⊔⊔⊔⊔
DAY: 18	⊔⊔⊔⊔⊔⊔⊔⊔
DAY: 19	⊔⊔⊔⊔⊔⊔⊔⊔
DAY: 20	⊔⊔⊔⊔⊔⊔⊔⊔
DAY: 21	⊔⊔⊔⊔⊔⊔⊔⊔
DAY: 22	⊔⊔⊔⊔⊔⊔⊔⊔
DAY: 23	⊔⊔⊔⊔⊔⊔⊔⊔
DAY: 24	⊔⊔⊔⊔⊔⊔⊔⊔
DAY: 25	⊔⊔⊔⊔⊔⊔⊔⊔
DAY: 26	⊔⊔⊔⊔⊔⊔⊔⊔
DAY: 27	⊔⊔⊔⊔⊔⊔⊔⊔
DAY: 28	⊔⊔⊔⊔⊔⊔⊔⊔
DAY: 29	⊔⊔⊔⊔⊔⊔⊔⊔
DAY: 30	⊔⊔⊔⊔⊔⊔⊔⊔

30 DAY WATER challenge

DAY: 1	DAY: 16
DAY: 2	DAY: 17
DAY: 3	DAY: 18
DAY: 4	DAY: 19
DAY: 5	DAY: 20
DAY: 6	DAY: 21
DAY: 7	DAY: 22
DAY: 8	DAY: 23
DAY: 9	DAY: 24
DAY: 10	DAY: 25
DAY: 11	DAY: 26
DAY: 12	DAY: 27
DAY: 13	DAY: 28
DAY: 14	DAY: 29
DAY: 15	DAY: 30

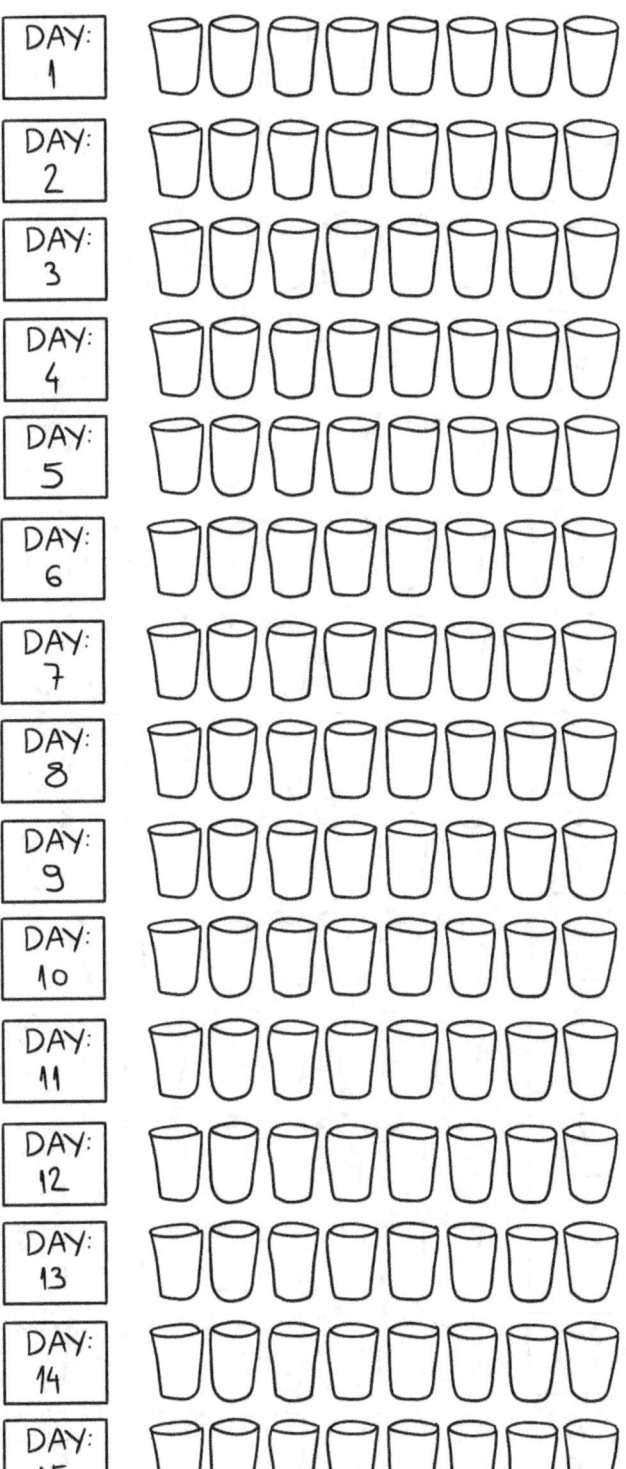

30 DAY
WATER
challenge

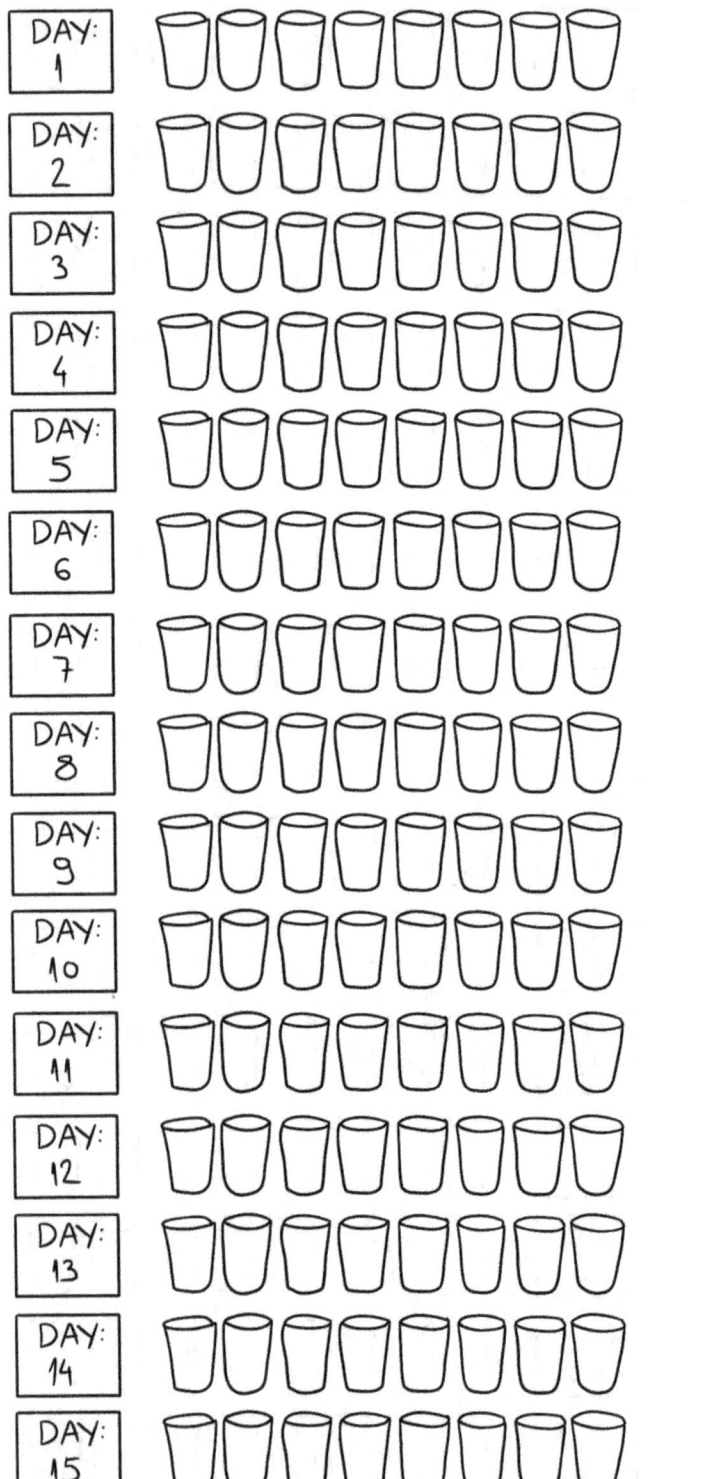

DAY: 1	DAY: 16
DAY: 2	DAY: 17
DAY: 3	DAY: 18
DAY: 4	DAY: 19
DAY: 5	DAY: 20
DAY: 6	DAY: 21
DAY: 7	DAY: 22
DAY: 8	DAY: 23
DAY: 9	DAY: 24
DAY: 10	DAY: 25
DAY: 11	DAY: 26
DAY: 12	DAY: 27
DAY: 13	DAY: 28
DAY: 14	DAY: 29
DAY: 15	DAY: 30

30 DAY
WATER
challenge

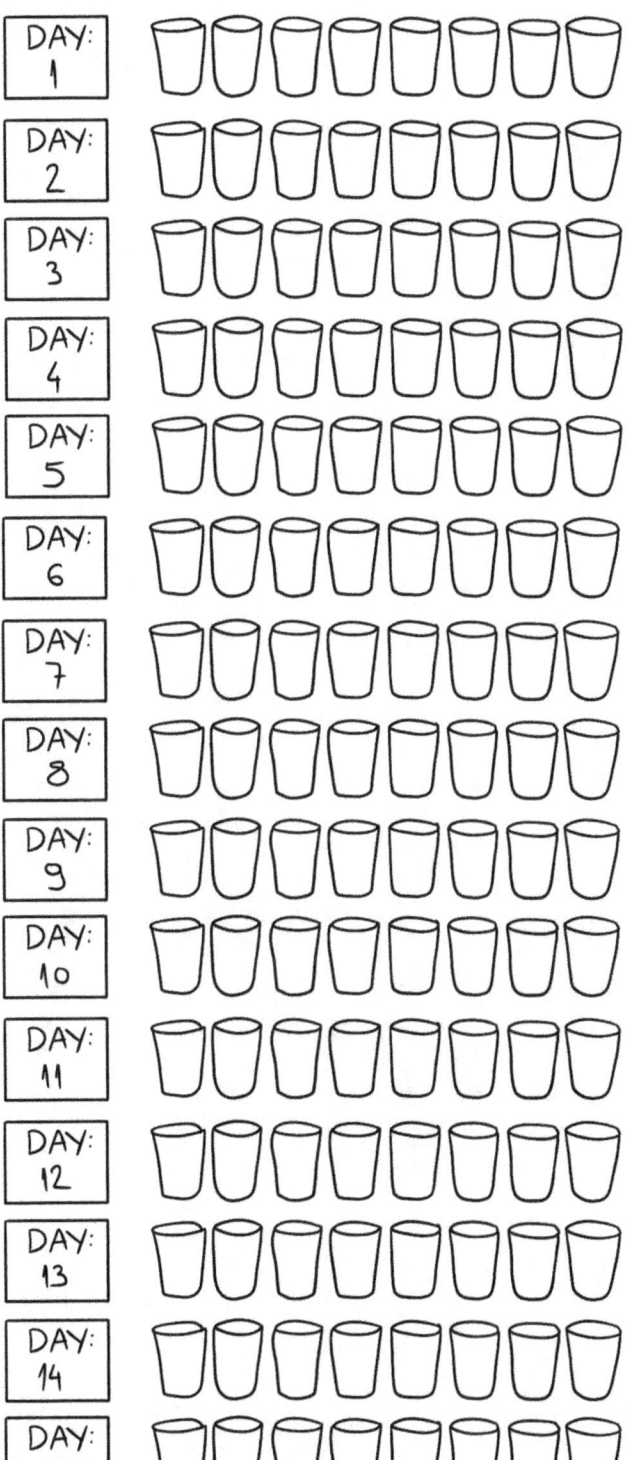

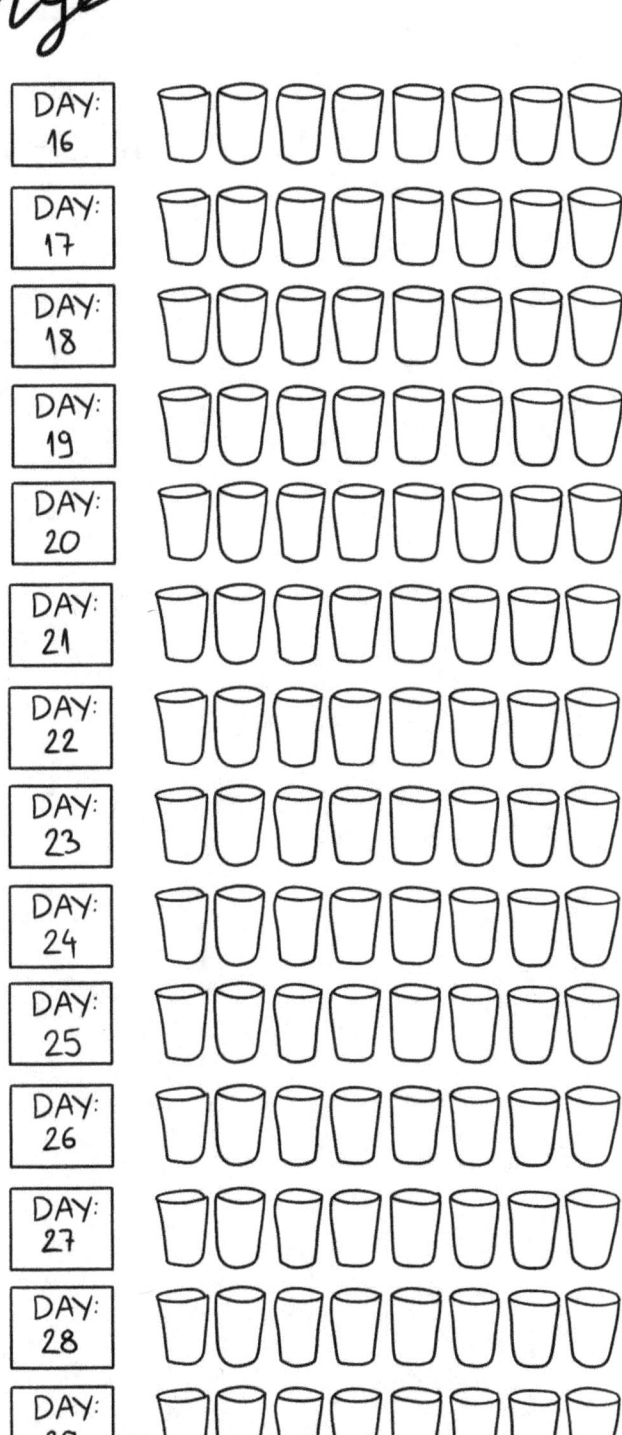

Takeaway notes:

_____

_____

_____

_____

_____

Year of use:

_____